PENGUIN BOOKS

EVA FRASER'S
FACE AND BODY PROGRAMME

Born in England in 1928, Eva Fraser grew up to be keenly interested in sport, and her first job was working as a tennis and squash instructor. She then went to work for one of London's top photographers, soon becoming involved in the more technical side of photographic printing.

She travelled widely, establishing a career in tapestry restoration, until a chance meeting in 1978 with Eva Hoffman. Madame Hoffman, then seventy-six years old, trained Eva in her facial exercise techniques, which she had devised with a doctor colleague in the 1930s. On her retirement, Madame Hoffman encouraged Eva to take over her work.

This method is taught in London in private one-to-one sessions. Through books and videos it is now available to a wider audience. Penguin also publish the bestselling *Eva Fraser's Facial Workout*

EVA FRASER'S
FACE AND BODY
PROGRAMME

PENGUIN BOOKS

To Eva Hoffmann

PENGUIN BOOKS

Published by the Penguin Group
Penguin Books Ltd, 27 Wrights Lane, London w8 5tz, England
Penguin Books USA Inc., 375 Hudson Street, New York, New York 10014, USA
Penguin Books Australia Ltd, Ringwood, Victoria, Australia
Penguin Books Canada Ltd, 10 Alcorn Avenue, Toronto, Ontario, Canada m4v 3b2
Penguin Books (NZ) Ltd, 182–190 Wairau Road, Auckland 10, New Zealand

Penguin Books Ltd, Registered Offices: Harmondsworth, Middlesex, England

First published by Viking 1992
Published in Penguin Books 1993
3 5 7 9 10 8 6 4

Printed in England by Clays Ltd, St Ives plc

CONTENTS

INTRODUCTION

When I opened my Facial Workout studio in London, I viewed my work as providing a keep-fit regime for the face. Within days, I realized this wasn't the main concern for many of my clients. Age and ageing were their main worries.

This subject became of great interest to me. Listening to both men and women discussing how they saw themselves and others was quite a revelation.

The age of a person is really quite irrelevant. I still can't view myself or others in terms simply of a number of years. I rarely ask anyone their age, it is just not that important – though most people do volunteer the information. The interesting thing is that very few people, of whatever age, think they are young. I have even found that this applies to people in their twenties.

At some time in our lives, ageing does become a concern for most of us. Eventually, this concern may pass as we gradually come to accept the process as inevitable. After all, what else can we do? However, I don't think this concern need necessarily trouble people any more. With the knowledge that the mind, spirit and body control our whole existence, we can – if we want – learn to regulate our lives so as to deal with many of the anxieties and fears we all encounter. The ageing process is just like everything else in this respect – it is a matter of noting what is happening and taking steps to put it right.

Occasionally, when talking about ageing, people say to me 'Oh Eva, it's all right for you.' Well, it isn't *all right* for anyone.

I have noticed that, although we all seem to have very

different 'joys' in life, we all have more or less the same anxieties. People feel that the fears they talk to me about are unique, but it's amazing how similar people's concerns appear to be, whatever their walk in life.

When it comes to age – and I don't mean ageing – a great deal has to be done to change our mental attitudes. Employers and the media don't help by being constantly preoccupied with youth – but this attitude *will* eventually change. In the meantime, it is most important to change our *own* attitudes and perceptions of age.

In my work, I so often hear, 'I'm afraid I'm not young – I'm nearly forty.' Only forty, for goodness' sake! How lucky can someone be? I think that some of us are really looking at ourselves in the wrong perspective. If we are comparing ourselves to how we were in our twenties, then of course we are older. But if we look at things differently and see ourselves as possibly living to be 100, then we must come to realize how young we are now.

Having said this, though, looking in the mirror each day and noting the gradual decline is not fun. But the decline need not be inevitable.

The main focus of my work is the face. With correct exercising, the improvement to the face can be amazing.

Thirteen years ago, I was as concerned about ageing as many others are today. Fortunately, I am concerned no more. I don't mean I have found the elixir of youth. Who has? Obviously, we will all age – but it is how we age and our attitudes to this that make all the difference.

Many of my clients now comment that they no longer *worry* about getting older. This is how I feel too, and this gives me a sense of freedom to get on with other things in life. Our mental attitude to age really does need to be positive. Many people never really appreciate the age they are at the time, and this goes on throughout their lives. When they are forty, they look back to being thirty; at fifty they long for the youthful days when they were forty; and so on. They always seem to be thinking ten years back and realizing how young they were *then*. This surely is missing out on life.

I suppose one of the reasons for attitudes like this is that there is nowadays so much emphasis on youth and physical perfection. It is almost as if ageing were a crime. In the USA, even teenagers are now undergoing cosmetic surgery to perfect their looks. These young girls obviously feel that if they are not the 'correct' fashionable shape of the moment then they are inadequate in some way. This is very sad, I think. Of course it is important to most of us to feel good and to look good, but how far should we go to keep up with changing standards of so-called beauty?

In spite of all the research, the mystery of ageing is still largely unsolved. We all age at different rates according to the changes in our cells, tissues and organs – and according to our mental attitudes too.

Here I could note down for you the symptoms of ageing we are likely to expect from the mid-forties onwards – but what would be the point? Some changes will happen sooner, some later, some never. Watching for them to happen is a pointless exercise.

Youth doesn't necessarily mean robust health, nor does old age necessarily mean illness and disability. In fact many people are healthier in later life than they were as children. To feel old through neglect of our bodies and minds is another matter, though, and that can happen at any age. Fortunately, however, the body has such recupera-tive powers that it can respond amazingly quickly to an overhaul even late in life.

Obviously, the earlier we start to look after ourselves the better. There is no point slowly committing suicide for forty years or more – smoking, drinking to excess, eating a poor diet – and then being surprised at the state of our health.

Expecting a doctor to cure our ills totally after years of neglect is unreasonable and a cure may not always be possible.

Fortunately, today there is so much on offer – so many alternative ways of revitalizing ourselves – that we have a huge choice. There are fitness courses at home or away, health spas, therapies for every ailment, alternative medicine – even the painful option of cosmetic surgery – the list is endless. Way up on my list, though, are body and facial exercises. They are the quickest, the safest (if you opt for a sensible regime) and the best way to reverse the signs of ageing and see an all-over improvement.

Everyone has their own ideas of fitness. The range here is very wide, depending on whether you are a professional athlete or just need sufficient fitness and strength for your everyday activities. But the fact is that anyone, if they so desire, can improve their appearance, well-being and mental powers whatever their circumstances or age.

Even taking every precaution imaginable, and barring accidents, the length of one's life is unknown. So the concern should really be: how well can I live from day to day? There is no doubt that the more we look after our basic needs – nutrition, mental and physical exercise and having fun – the more chance we have of staying fit and healthy, hopefully throughout our lives.

Wanting to extend life, to live to 100 years or more, makes no sense to me. In most things, the length of time is irrelevant. Measured in time alone, life, love, friendships, careers mean very little. The important thing, I feel, is what they really mean at the time. Knowing someone you really love continues for ever. It has nothing to do with how long you have known them. Being married for fifty years or more, or having the same job for most of your working life, may be admirable, but it means nothing, if you haven't enjoyed it, if you haven't given of your best.

I believe that most of us have a choice about the way we

live out our time on earth – at least in the Western world – although it often doesn't seem so. We all feel driven or pressured at times, but if we stop and think we realize that we seldom really are.

It is a comforting day-dream to imagine 'If it wasn't for him or her or the government or whatever, I would have been . . .' In fact we have far more control over our own fate than that attitude implies. Subconsciously, we do choose what we need, or perhaps what we can cope with, in our lives. Maybe from time to time, we should consider whether we need reprogramming. It is all too easy to go on, year after year, being too busy to look at one's life and take stock of it. It is a good idea occasionally to stop and consider what it is you need in order to lead a more fulfilling life for yourself and for those around you.

Everyone needs to give themselves space and time for the things they want to do. This isn't selfish – it is an absolute necessity. For myself, I have found periods of retreat essential throughout my life. Not just holidays, but a semi-withdrawal from the outside world – to just stop; to walk among trees; to cease talking for once and recuperate. I don't only love these times, I find them essential.

This may all sound very self-indulgent. Surely there is more to life, more going on out there in the world, than this? Well, of course there is. However, if you don't help yourself – get yourself sorted out from time to time – then it is very difficult to feel free to help others. Just by feeling happier in yourself, you can affect everyone around you. And it is your own responsibility to see that your everyday surroundings and contacts are as pleasing as possible.

It is certainly true that our relationships have a great deal to do with our well-being. Working or living with people we are not happy with must inevitably affect our health. Working each day with no enthusiasm for the job surely must be soul-destroying.

Many of us have responsibilities that make any dramatic change in our lives impossible. However, if a complete change is not possible, we can always rearrange things.

It is possible to rearrange relationships, by concentrating on what you like about someone instead of searching for the things you don't like. This invariably leads to a better understanding.

If you are tired of where you live but are unable to move, then rearrange the rooms, the furniture, the decor.

If you are not happy with your appearance, then consider what it is you could change about that. Your hairstyle perhaps, or your make-up. Would you be happier if you were thinner or fatter? Do you need a different style in clothes? If you are not very good at this, advice from a colour and wardrobe consultant is a good idea. Alternatively, involve a friend whose advice you trust and have some fun.

Are you tired of your marriage? Perhaps you need more friends in your life, more outside interests, so that you and your partner have more to discuss together. Maybe you need to give more love.

It is important to look at any situation that isn't working as you would like and see what you can do to improve things. Very often all that's needed is quite a small adjustment. Any one can take charge, at any time they choose and build for themselves the environment they desire.

Just making resolutions – New Year or otherwise – seldom produces results. I think a better way is to decide which is the *one* thing that would bring you more happiness and fulfilment in your life. Having decided, go all out to make it happen. Live it, dream it, have total enthusiasm for it and – most important of all – take action. If you want it enough, you can make almost anything happen. It is essential for your well-being to find the one thing that can make your life more worthwhile.

It is seldom considered that depression, tiredness or even illness may simply be caused by boredom – not necessarily through having too little to do but through lack of variety in your everyday activities. This can apply to people in any walk of life, whether confined to the home or out at work.

Fear of failure is often an obstacle to doing new things, but failure can be just as rewarding as success. We all know the rewards of success, but, if looked at as a learning process, failure can be very stimulating too. Obviously if failure happens too often then you are on the wrong track, but otherwise it can be a great incentive to replan and start again.

Many of us forget how important it is to congratulate ourselves on things we do well. Be aware of these and give yourself a pat on the back from time to time. You can feel very deflated waiting for other people to notice things you do. Instead, if you have done something well, you should feel delighted irrespective of others. Small achievements are just as important as big ones – even clearing out a cupboard that you have meant to tackle for ages. You can apply this principle to many things in your everyday life. It is all too easy to feel that you never achieve anything, but that simply isn't true.

Being interested in life, having a sense of humour, not taking yourself too seriously, your state of mind – all these add up to make you what you are. Being outwardly beautiful can be an added bonus, but fortunately it is not the most important thing. We all know people we love to be with, whom we just feel happy around, and their looks or age have nothing to do with this feeling.

Every age has its attractions. For example, retirement should mean a chance to do all, or at least some, of the things you may have been wanting to do for years but never had the time for. If this eventually means sitting about the house, gardening, watching television and very little else – well, that is one option.

Another option is to take this time, which could in fact be considerable – as much as thirty years – and use it to study or to travel, to start a new career or to pursue a pastime that you can now concentrate on to your heart's content. It can be a very exciting time – possibly the most exciting time of your life.

My oldest client was eighty-two when we first met and had just sold her catering business, which provided picnic hampers. Since then she has learned how to hand-paint screens, and this is now her flourishing career at eighty-four years old. Her huge enthusiasm and zest for life are fantastic and very inspiring.

State of mind and awareness are both important in everything we do in life. Being helpful to others whenever you can; being aware of the help others give you – just small things like opening doors and letting others go first – these are all giving love and care, however trivial they seem.

As you read on, you will come across ideas and practical ways of building on your own personal assets. Don't try and do everything at once. Consider what is most important to you *now*, and start there.

My thanks go to:
Marion, my partner; my many clients and friends; Oliver; Emily, Tamsin, Marion and Liz – the perfect models; and Clare Alexander and all at Viking, for their hard work and enthusiasm.

THE FOUR-WEEK FACIAL EXERCISE PLAN

The following Facial Workout programme has been devised to give you an easy-to-follow facial exercise plan. It is an accelerated, intensive version of the programme in my previous book, *Eva Fraser's Facial Workout*, that can give visible results in only four weeks.

The exercises are divided into four stages. Each group of exercises should be performed for one week. Even after the first week you should be able to feel a difference in your facial muscles, and by the time you have completed the fourth week you'll be well on your way to a more youthful you, and a lifetime's enjoyable facial exercising!

However, those of you who have not encountered the Facial Workout method before may find that one week at each stage is not enough. If so, *don't worry* and, above all, *don't give up*. What is most important is to learn the exercises carefully and thoroughly, and to practise them frequently and regularly. Take whatever time you need and get to know the workings of your facial muscles. Results may only be gradual, as the muscles take time to strengthen and build, but with steady, daily application you *will* soon start to see the difference.

Anyone who wishes to master the original Workout in its complete form should refer to my previous book, *Eva Fraser's Facial Workout*. But for those of you who have mastered the facial exercises already, the exercise plan outlined here will provide the perfect refresher course.

THE MUSCLES OF THE FACE

Before starting the Facial Workout routines, it is worth briefly studying the facial-muscles chart on the opposite page. It is intriguing to visualize what is going on under our skin.

Contrary to what many people think, the facial muscles get very little exercise. In fact, they get no exercise at all in the true sense – they simply cause movement. It's as though you think you have exercised the body by simply standing up and sitting down. Of course this is movement, but it is far from a workout that will keep you in good shape.

In order to keep your facial contour in shape, you do need to work out in a positive way. The *only* way to strengthen muscles, whether of the face or the body, is through exercise.

Lines on the face are not necessarily caused by ageing, unless they are very deep. (These ingrained lines are usually caused by overexposure to the sun and deterioration of the collagen fibres that hold the muscles together.) Very young people frequently have lines on their faces, and yet they usually look no older than their years. It is really the drooping and sagging of the facial muscles that has such an ageing effect. If you have ever had someone say 'Cheer up' to you when you were in fact feeling perfectly happy, this may be a sign that your facial muscles need strengthening. This can be done, but only by a regular workout for these muscles.

Some creams can improve skin texture, but they do nothing to strengthen the muscles, whether of the body or of the face.

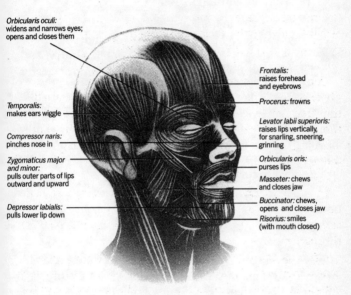

Orbicularis oculi:
widens and narrows eyes;
opens and closes them

Temporalis:
makes ears wiggle

Compressor naris:
pinches nose in

*Zygomaticus major
and minor:*
pulls outer parts of lips
outward and upward

Depressor labialis:
pulls lower lip down

Frontalis:
raises forehead
and eyebrows

Procerus: frowns

Levator labii superioris:
raises lips vertically,
for snarling, sneering,
grinning

Orbicularis oris:
purses lips

Masseter: chews
and closes jaw

Buccinator: chews,
opens and closes jaw

Risorius: smiles
(with mouth closed)

PREPARATION

Your Facial Workout programme must be followed with total relaxed concentration.

- Always exercise in front of a mirror.
- Always watch and concentrate on every movement.
- Always choose a time when you are not in a hurry.
- Always exercise with a clean skin – no make-up or creams.

You may find it helpful to use Vaseline to lubricate the under-eye area *only*, but never use eye creams or eye gels for this purpose. Apply the Vaseline with the pads of your middle fingers, starting at your temples and *very lightly* smoothing downwards then under your eyes towards the bridge of your nose.

RELAXATION

Always begin your programme in a relaxed state, preferably in a warm room, on your own. Put a 'Do Not Disturb' sign on the door if necessary – you will get nowhere if people are always coming in and out. Set aside a time for yourself.

Sit in front of your mirror.

Now close your eyes and completely relax.

Visualize a beautiful scene, perhaps a place you know where you feel happy – a meadow, the mountains, a garden – wherever you feel at peace.

Slowly breathe in and out – naturally.

When you are ready, open your eyes and start your programme.

FACIAL WORKOUT – STAGE 1

The first six exercises in this section consist of a warm-up routine. They will accustom you to locating and moving the muscles of your face and get you ready for the more advanced stages of your course.

Please take your time over this first stage – it is of para-mount importance.

To give you more awareness of the muscle movement, you may at first find it easier to touch the face *lightly* with your fingertips in the direction of the arrows on the illustrations.

Do *not*, however, assist the movement with your fingers.

In each exercise, every movement must start from the point specified.

The skin under the eyes will form creases as you smile up. However, do not squint or tense your eye muscles.

WARM-UP EXERCISE 1

Sit in front of a mirror.

Keep your back teeth lightly together, *without tension*, lips slightly apart.

1 In five slow movements, smile very slowly in the direction of the arrows on the illustration, to the mid-ear position.
Hold for a count of five after each movement.

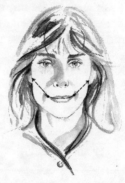

2 Return slowly to the starting position, in five slow movements with counts of five between.

Do this three times.

> *Each movement must be felt as a lift of the muscle, without tension.*

WARM-UP EXERCISE 2

Sit in front of a mirror.

Keep your back teeth lightly together, *without tension*, lips slightly apart.

1 In five slow movements, smile very slowly towards your temples. Each time, feel a good 'lift' from the position of the dots on the illustration. Hold for a count of five after each movement.

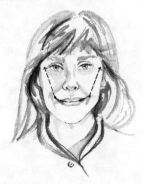

2 Return slowly to the starting position, in five slow movements with counts of five between.

Do this three times.

> *Throughout this exercise, be sure to keep your eye muscles relaxed.*
> *Do not squint.*

WARM-UP EXERCISE 3

Sit in front of a mirror

Keep your back teeth lightly together, *without tension*, lips slightly apart.

> *With your fingertips, lightly stroke each side of your face in the direction of the arrows on the illustration, for awareness of the movement. Do not, however, assist the movement with your fingers.*

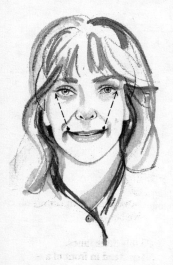

1 In five slow movements, smile up very slowly towards your outer eye corners. Each time, feel a good 'lift' from the position of the dots on the illustration.
Hold for a count of five after each movement.

2 Return slowly to the starting position, in five slow movements with counts of five between.

Do this three times.

> *Throughout this exercise, be sure to keep your eye muscles relaxed. Do not squint.*

16

WARM-UP EXERCISE 4

Sit in front of a mirror

Keep your back teeth lightly together, *without tension*, lips slightly apart.

> *Again, you may find it easier to touch the face very lightly with your fingertips, for awareness of the movement of the muscles throughout this exercise. An inch or so out from the nostrils on each side is a good position. Do not press or assist the movement with your fingers – it's your facial muscles that have to do all the work.*

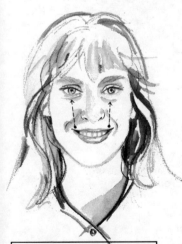

1 In five slow movements, smile up very slowly towards the centre of your eyes. Each time, feel a good 'lift' from the position of the dots on the illustration.
Hold for a count of five after each movement.

2 Return slowly to the starting position, in five slow movements with counts of five between.

Do this three times.
Sit or stand in front of a mirror.

> *Throughout this exercise, be sure to keep your eye muscles relaxed.*
> *Do not squint.*

WARM-UP EXERCISE 5

Sit in front of a mirror.

Keep your back teeth lightly together, *without tension*, lips
slightly apart.

1 In five slow movements, raise the muscles
   on both sides of your nostrils in the
   direction of the arrows on the illustration.
   These movements are like a gradual snarl.
   Hold for a count of five after each
   movement.

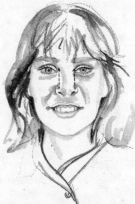

2 Return slowly to the starting position,
   in five slow movements with counts of
   five between.

Do this three times.

> *Throughout this exercise, be sure to keep*
> *your eye muscles relaxed.*
> *Do not squint.*

WARM-UP EXERCISE 6

Sit in front of a mirror.

Relax completely.

1 Raise your eyebrows very slowly in
five slow movements.
Really stretch up with your eyebrows
in the fifth movement.

2 With your eyes *wide* open, hold for a
count of five.

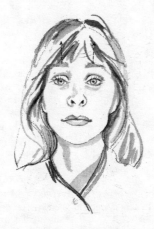

3 Slowly lower your eyebrows to the
starting position, in five slow
movements.

Close your eyes. Relax and breathe.

Do this three times.

TO FIRM MUSCLES UNDER THE CHIN AND HELP ELIMINATE A DOUBLE CHIN

Sit in front of a mirror.

> *Don't hold your fist too firmly against your chin.*

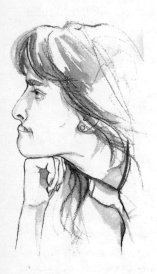

> *Don't squint –*
> *keep your eyes relaxed.*
> *Close your eyes if preferred.*

1 Your mouth should be closed and your jaw relaxed. Jut your chin forward and *very slightly* upwards.

2 Rest your elbow on a table. Place your clenched fist under your chin as a gentle resistance. Slide your lower lip up and over your top lip, towards your nose.

3 Now press the *tip* of your tongue against the roof of your mouth, just behind your top teeth. Gradually increase the pressure during a count of five. The *tip* of your tongue should do all the work.

4 Wait for a few seconds, then slowly release the pressure during a count of five.

Relax and breathe.

Do this three times.

If you find the exercises in Stage 1 easy to do – if you are able to feel your facial muscles beginning to come alive – then, and only then, continue to Stage 2. Otherwise, work through Stage 1 exercises for a little longer.

FACIAL WORKOUT – STAGE 2

You may now discontinue the exercises in Stage 1.

The warm-up exercises in Stage 2 are very similar to those in Stage 1, except that you are now working the muscles on only *one side* of the face at a time. At this stage you are still learning to locate and control your facial muscles.

So do the next five exercises moving the muscles on the *right-hand side* of your face only.

Then repeat the exercises moving the muscles on the *left-hand side* of your face only.

One side is usually weaker than the other, so you may find these movements a little difficult at first. Keep going though – your muscles will gradually become stronger.

It is important to work out regularly, on five or six days a week at first. This will give you really good results. When you have completed this programme and your facial muscles have strengthened, then three times a week – about ten minutes each time – will be sufficient to keep them in shape.

WARM-UP EXERCISE 1

Sit in front of a mirror.

Keep your back teeth lightly together, *without tension*, lips slightly apart.

1 In five slow movements with the right-hand corner of your mouth *only*, smile very slowly in the direction of the arrow on the illustration to the mid-ear position.
Hold for a count of five after each movement.

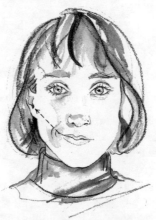

2 Return slowly to the starting position, in five slow movements with counts of five between.

Each movement must be felt as a lift of the muscle, without tension.

WARM-UP EXERCISE 2

Sit in front of a mirror.

Keep your back teeth lightly together, *without tension*, lips slightly apart.

1 In five slow movements with the right-hand corner of your mouth *only*, smile up very slowly towards your temple. Each time, feel a good 'lift' from the position of the dot on the illustration.
Hold for a count of five after each movement.

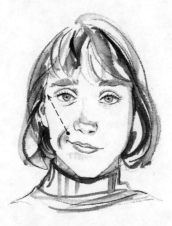

2 Return slowly to the starting position, in five slow movements with counts of five between.

Do not squint or tense your eye muscles.

WARM-UP EXERCISE 3

Sit in front of a mirror.

Keep your back teeth lightly together, *without tension*, lips slightly apart.

1 In five slow movements with the right-hand corner of your mouth *only*, smile up very slowly towards your outer eye corner. Each time, feel a good 'lift' from the position of the dot on the illustration.
Hold for a count of five after each movement.

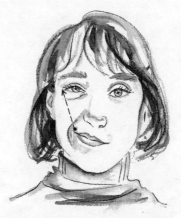

2 Return slowly to the starting position, in five slow movements with counts of five between.

Do not squint or tense your eye muscles.

WARM-UP EXERCISE 4

Sit in front of a mirror.

Keep your back teeth lightly together, *without tension*, lips slightly apart.

1 In five slow movements with the right-hand corner of your mouth *only*, smile up very slowly towards the centre of your eye. Each time, feel a good 'lift' from the position of the dot on the illustration.
Hold for a count of five after each movement.

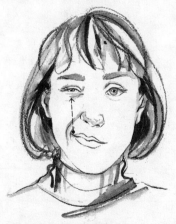

2 Return slowly to the starting position, in five slow movements with counts of five between.

Do not squint or tense your eye muscles.

WARM-UP EXERCISE 5

Sit in front of a mirror.

Keep your back teeth lightly together, *without tension*, lips
slightly apart.

1   In five slow movements, raise the
muscle on the right side of your
nostrils *only* in the direction of the
arrow on the illustration. These
movements are like a gradual snarl.
Hold for a count of five after each
movement.

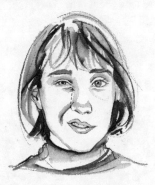

> *Do not squint or tense your eye muscles.*

2   Return slowly to the starting position,
in five slow movements with counts of
five between.

You have performed the last five exercises on *one side* of your
face only.
Now repeat the exercises using the muscles on the other side of the
face, relaxing and breathing frequently throughout these routines.

WARM-UP EXERCISE 6

Sit in front of a mirror.

Relax completely.

1 Raise your eyebrows very slowly in
   five slow movements. Really stretch
   up with your eyebrows in the fifth
   movement.

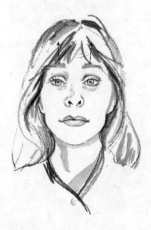

2 With your eyes *wide* open, hold for a
   count of five.

3 Slowly lower your eyebrows to the
   starting position, in five slow
   movements.

Close your eyes. Relax and breathe.

Do this three times.

TO STRENGTHEN THE MUSCLES OF THE UPPER CHEEKS

For this exercise, apply Vaseline on the under-eye area – do not use eye creams or gels.

> *Here again you may find it easier to touch the face very lightly with your fingertips, for awareness of the movement of the muscles throughout this exercise. Do not press or assist the movement with your fingers. Your facial muscles must do all the work, so no pushing please.*

Sit or stand in front of a mirror.

Keep your back teeth lightly together, *without tension*, lips slightly apart.

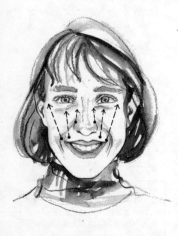

1 In five slow movements, lift all the muscles in the direction of the arrows on the illustration. Feel all these muscles lifting simultaneously. Every upward movement starts from the position of the dots on the illustration. After each lifting movement, pause for a count of five.

2 Return slowly to the starting position, in five slow movements with counts of five between.

Do this three times.

> *Do not squint or tense your eye muscles.*

TO WORK THE MUSCLES OF THE NECK AND JAW LINE

Leave this exercise out if you have any jaw problems.

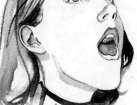

Sit or stand in front of a mirror.

1 With a straight spine, tilt your head up and back slightly. Now jut out your chin.

2 In this position, keeping head still, open your mouth widely by lowering your jaw. Now grin widely.

3 Bring your back teeth together gently. Now – still grinning – lower and raise your jaw ten times.

Relax and breathe.

Do this only once.

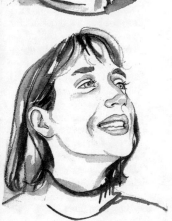

DOS
Keep the wide grin position throughout. Concentrate on the lifting of the jaw.

DON'TS
Do not gnash your teeth together. There should be no tension in your forehead. There should be no tension in your eye area.

TO FIRM MUSCLES UNDER THE CHIN AND HELP ELIMINATE A DOUBLE CHIN

Don't hold your fist too firmly against your chin.

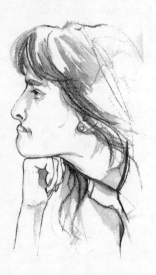

*Don't squint –
keep your eyes relaxed.
Close your eyes if preferred.*

Sit in front of a mirror.

1 Your mouth should be closed and your jaw relaxed. Jut your chin forward and *very slightly* upwards.

2 Rest your elbow on a table. Place your clenched fist under your chin as a gentle resistance. Slide your lower lip up and over your top lip, towards your nose.

3 Now press the *tip* of your tongue against the roof of your mouth, just behind your top teeth. Gradually increase the pressure during a count of five. The *tip* of your tongue should do all the work.

4 Wait for a few seconds, then slowly release the pressure during a count of five.

Relax and breathe.

Do this three times.

At this stage you should feel quite a difference in the tone of your facial muscles. You will need to feel this improvement before you go on to the next stage.

FACIAL WORKOUT – STAGE 3

You may now discontinue the exercises in Stage 2.

Stage 3 of the Facial Workout begins with an exercise from the previous stage.

You should start with this exercise whenever you do your Facial Workout – it is an excellent warm-up exercise before any facial programme.

For some of the exercises that follow you will need a pair of cotton gloves, to prevent your fingerhold from slipping and to prevent damage by your fingernails.

TO STRENGTHEN THE MUSCLES OF THE UPPER CHEEKS

For this exercise, apply Vaseline on the under-eye area – do not use eye creams or gels.

Sit or stand in front of a mirror.

Keep your back teeth lightly together, *without tension*, lips slightly apart.

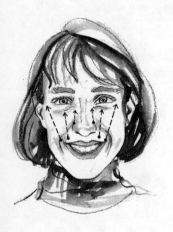

1 In five slow movements, lift all the muscles in the direction of the arrows on the illustration. Feel all these muscles lifting simultaneously. Every upward movement starts from the position of the dots on the illustration. After each lifting movement, pause for a count of five.

2 Return slowly to the starting position, in five slow movements with counts of five between.

Do this three times.

As you perform this exercise, the skin under the eyes will go into creases – this is quite normal. However, do not squint or tense your eye muscles. Keeping your eyes wide open will help avoid this.

TO HELP ELIMINATE JOWLS AND IMPROVE THE JAW LINE AND NECK

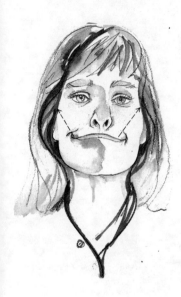

Sit or stand in front of a mirror.

1 Jut your chin upwards so that the front of your neck is held taut.

2 Slide your lower lip over your top lip, as far up towards your nose as possible.

3 With a stretched feeling in the front of your neck, slowly smile up and outwards in the direction of the arrows during a count of five.

4 Hold for a slow count of five while stroking upwards on the jaw line with the flat of your fingers and palms.

5 Return slowly to the starting position during a count of five. Gradually release your lip hold.

Relax and breathe.

Do this three times.

You should feel a good pull around your jaw line and throat.

TO ELIMINATE HORIZONTAL LINES ON THE FOREHEAD

Sit in front of a mirror.

1 Rest your elbows on a table and place the pads of your fingertips along your hairline, on the points marked with dots on the illustration.

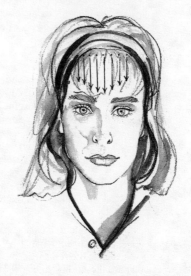

> *All the movements must come from the top of the forehead downwards.*

2 Gently push your brow upwards and hold it against the bone.

TO ELIMINATE HORIZONTAL LINES
ON THE FOREHEAD

Do not scowl.

*Do not push your head into your hands –
this will cause tension at the back of your
neck.*

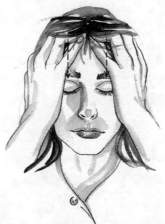

3 With head erect, look straight ahead.
   Now try to bring your brow down in
   five movements against the resistance
   of your hold, gradually closing your
   eyes.

4 Hold this downward pull for a count
   of three, then slowly release.

Relax and breathe.

Do this three times.

TO STRENGTHEN THE LOWER CHEEK MUSCLES

Wearing cotton gloves, sit or stand in front of a mirror.

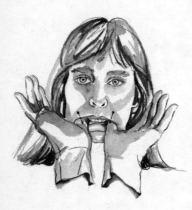

1 Place your thumbs inside your mouth, between your back teeth and your cheeks. Your thumb-nails should face your back teeth; your palms should face upwards.

2 Hold your thumbs rigidly ½ inch away from your teeth.

3 In eight small movements, pull back your cheek muscles against the resistance of your thumbs.

4 Hold for a count of five.

5 Return slowly to the starting position, in eight small movements.

Relax and breathe.

Do this three times.

Do not squint or scowl during this exercise.

TO STRENGTHEN THE UPPER EYELIDS

Lack of exercise can cause the eyelids to droop considerably, making the eyes look smaller and the lids go into folds with drooping corners. Working the eyelid muscles can give a much more youthful and alert appearance.

Sit or stand looking *straight ahead* into a mirror throughout this exercise.

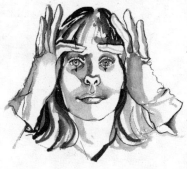

1 Curve your index fingers under your eyebrows.

2 Push up your eyebrows and hold them against the bone. It is important to keep this firm hold throughout.

3 Close your eyelids very slowly, feeling a good downward pull from brow to lashes.

4 Now squeeze your eyelids together really tightly. Hold for a count of five.

5 Release the squeeze slowly during a count of five.

6 Open your eyes. Relax and breathe.

Do this three times.

Be careful not to scowl during this exercise. The muscle movement must come straight downwards in the direction of the cheeks.

TO STRENGTHEN THE UNDER-EYE MUSCLES

Strengthening the under-eye muscles will help to eliminate lines, bags and puffiness.

For this exercise, apply Vaseline on the under-eye area – do not use eye creams or gels.

You may find it easier to do this exercise standing in front of a mirror. Lean towards the mirror, with your hands resing on a table or wash-basin to steady you.

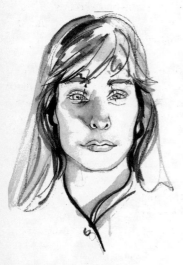

Watch your eyes in the mirror – do not blink.

1 Raise your eyebrows fractionally. Then slowly raise your lower lids, in five small movements. The muscle movement goes upwards, towards the bridge of the nose.

2 Close your eyes gently and squeeze the lids together. Hold this squeeze for a count of five, then slowly relax the squeeze.

3 With your eyes still closed, slowly release the lower lid muscles, in five slow movements.

4 Open your eyes. Relax and breathe.

Do this three times.

> *Be careful not to scowl. Remember to lift the lower lids until almost shut before closing your eyes.*

FACIAL WORKOUT – STAGE 4

One of the things that most causes the face to look old is slackening of the upper cheeks. However, through exercise, this condition can be reversed – giving once again a more alive, youthful appearance.

In order to work these muscles properly, it is necessary at first to get them moving in a simple way – to be aware of them. That was the point of the warm-up exercises in the earlier sections. It is important to have really prepared these muscles before starting this section.

In some of the following exercises you will be working the muscles against the resistance of a hold. You may find this difficult at first, but, I promise you, with practice, it does become quite easy. In fact difficulties can be caused by 'trying too hard'.

It is important:
● to feel relaxed;
● *not* to tense the muscles – this includes the muscles of forehead, eyes, neck, shoulders and even the feet;
● to really concentrate on each movement of the muscles.

You will need a pair of cotton gloves, to prevent your fingerhold from slipping and to prevent damage by your fingernails.

Alternatively you could use some fine towelling, or two cotton handkerchiefs, or even two tissues – but not if your skin is very sensitive.

Like Stage 3, this section of the exercise routine begins with the upper-cheek exercise you have come across earlier.

TO STRENGTHEN THE MUSCLES OF THE UPPER CHEEKS

For this exercise, apply Vaseline on the under-eye area – do not use eye creams or gels.

Sit or stand in front of a mirror.
Keep your back teeth lightly together, *without tension*, lips slightly apart.

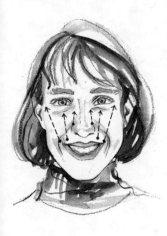

1 In five slow movements, lift all the muscles in the direction of the arrows on the illustration. Feel all these muscles lifting simultaneously. Every upward movement starts from the position of the dots on the illustration. After each lifting movement, pause for a count of five.

2 Return slowly to the starting position, in five slow movements with counts of five between.

You need do this only once here, then start the three-part upper-cheek exercises.

Here again you may find it easier to touch the face very lightly with your fingertips, for awareness of the movement of the muscles throughout this exercise. Do not press or assist the movement with your fingers. Your facial muscles must do all the work, so no pushing please.

TO BUILD AND STRENGTHEN THE UPPER CHEEK MUSCLES – STAGE 1

Building and strengthening the upper cheek muscles will give a fuller, high-cheekbone appearance.

Wearing cotton gloves, sit in front of a mirror, with your elbows resting on a table.

1 Place the flats of your thumbs in each side of your mouth, between your back teeth and your cheeks. Your thumb-nails should be facing your teeth and pointing towards the tops of your ears.

2 Hold on outside with the side of your curved index fingers. Your palms should be facing towards the mirror, as shown in the illustration.

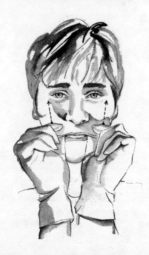

TO BUILD AND STRENGTHEN THE UPPER CHEEK MUSCLES – STAGE 1

3 Curve your thumbs slightly forward. Keep your hands steady and hold them down slightly.

4 In five slow movements, lift your upper cheek muscles in the direction of the arrows. Each lift must start from the holding position. Pause for a count of five after each movement.

5 Return to the starting position, in five slow movements with counts of five between.

Relax and breathe.

Do this three times.

> *When you start this Workout, only lift in two movements. Gradually increase the number of lifts to five as you are able to.*
>
> *Do not squint or tense your eye muscles. You may find it easier to keep your eyes wide open here.*

TO BUILD AND STRENGTHEN THE UPPER CHEEK MUSCLES – STAGE 2

Wearing cotton gloves, sit in front of a mirror, with your elbows resting on a table.

1 Place the flats of your thumbs in each side of your mouth, between your teeth and your cheeks. Your thumbnails should be facing your teeth; your thumbs should be pointing towards the outer eye corners.

2 Hold on outside with the side of your curved index fingers, with your knuckles facing each other.

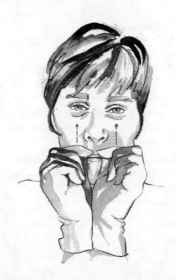

TO BUILD AND STRENGTHEN THE
UPPER CHEEK MUSCLES – STAGE 2

3 Curve your thumbs slightly forward. Keep your hands steady and hold them down slightly.

4 In five slow movements, lift your upper cheek muscles in the direction of the arrows. Each lift must start from the holding position. Pause for a count of five after each movement.

5 Return to the starting position, in five slow movements with counts of five between.

Relax and breathe.

Do this three times.

Start this Workout with only two upward lifts. Gradually increase the number of lifts to five as you are able to.

Do not squint or tense your eye muscles.

TO BUILD AND STRENGTHEN THE UPPER CHEEK MUSCLES – STAGE 3

Wearing cotton gloves, sit in front of a mirror, with your elbows resting on a table.

1 Place the flats of your thumbs in each side of your mouth, between your teeth and your cheeks. Your thumbnails should be facing your teeth; your thumbs should be pointing towards the inner eye corners.

2 Hold on outside with the side of your curved index fingers, with your knuckles facing and touching each other.

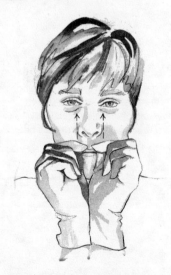

TO BUILD AND STRENGTHEN THE
UPPER CHEEK MUSCLES – STAGE 3

3 Curve your thumbs slightly forward. Keep your hands steady and hold them down slightly.

4 In three slow movements, lift the muscles each side of your nose against the resistance of your hold. Pause for a count of five after each movement.

5 Return to the starting position, in three slow movements with counts of five between.

Relax and breathe.

Do this three times.

Never allow your hand/finger resistance to move up with the muscle lift. You are working the muscles against the hold.

Do not squint or tense your eye muscles.

Do not scowl.

TO STRENGTHEN THE LIPS AND THE SURROUNDING MUSCLES

Sit or stand. Look into a mirror. Feel relaxed.

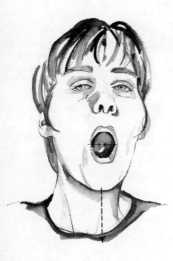

1 Open your mouth slightly as if to yawn (about a 1-inch gap).

2 Now lower your jaw in eight slow movements, at the same time gradually moving the corners of your mouth inwards.

After the eighth movement your mouth must form an *oval* (not a round) shape. Your lips and surrounding areas should feel very taut at this stage, with your jaw dropped down as far as possible.

3 Hold this position for a count of five. Then relax your *top lip* in eight slow movements to return to the starting position.

Relax and breathe.

Do this three times.

TO ELIMINATE LINES ON THE UPPER LIP

Wearing cotton gloves, rest your elbows on a table and look into a mirror.

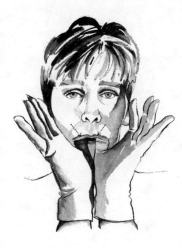

1 Place your thumbs under your top lip, with your thumb-nails resting against your gums. Your thumbs should point towards the centre of your eyes.

2 Now, feeling very relaxed, gently move your upper lip muscles towards your thumbs in eight small movements.

3 With your upper lip muscles very firmly pressed against your thumbs, hold for a count of five.

4 Keeping your thumbs in the same position, release your muscles in eight slow movements.

Relax and breathe.

Do this three times.

The space between your thumbs must remain the same throughout.

TO STRENGTHEN THE LOWER LIP AND THE CHIN MUSCLES

Wearing cotton gloves, look into a mirror.

Keep your teeth about 1 inch apart.

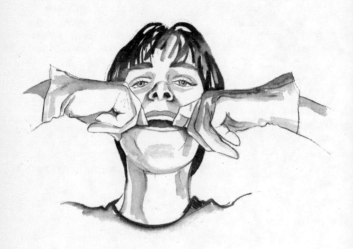

1 Hook the first joint of your index fingers behind your lower lip, with your finger-nails slightly away from your lower teeth and gums.

2 Move your lower lip's muscles against your finger resistance, in eight small movements.

TO STRENGTHEN THE LOWER LIP
AND THE CHIN MUSCLES

3 With your muscles very firmly pressed
against your fingers, hold for a count
of five.

4 Keeping your fingers in the same
position, release your muscles in eight
small movements.

Relax and breathe.

Do this three times.

> *Finger resistance must remain constant
> throughout.*
>
> *Keep the finger pressure in a slightly upward
> direction, to prevent a crease between the
> lower lip and chin.*

TO SLIM AND SHAPE THE LOWER CHEEKS

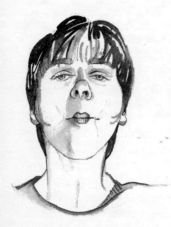

Sit or stand in front of a mirror.

1 Breathe two or three times.

2 Lift chin up and out.

3 Now suck your cheeks in for a count of ten.

Relax and breathe.

Do this three times.

Keep your eyes open.
Do not squint or scowl.

This completes your four-stage exercise plan.

You can repeat these sessions indefinitely – at first, once a day on five or six days a week; later, two or three times a week.

It isn't necessary to repeat the warm-up routines, unless you wish to do so from time to time.

I personally prefer to work out for about five minutes every other day, doing the exercises I feel I need at the time. However, you should do this only when you feel you have 'built' your facial muscles sufficiently.

On page 53 you will see a section on skin care, with a facial toning regime. Please try to follow this regime daily – or at least three times a week. It really is important for your skin and muscle tone and texture.

SKIN CARE

There are so many different preparations and so many schools of thought on what is the best form of skin care that it is easy to become confused about which is the best approach for *you*. No one can lay down rules for everyone, so choosing your personal skin-care routine has to be partly a matter of trial and error.

When you try out any skin-care product or regime, it is essential that you keep track of what is actually happening. There is no point in continuing to apply a face cream that promises you dramatically wonderful results, say, if from day to day you see it having the opposite effect. It may be difficult not to go on using a beauty preparation on which you have spent a lot of money; nevertheless, it is absurd to carry on with *anything* that is having an adverse effect just because you have paid for it. Throw it away!

In my opinion, facial exercises are the great face-savers of all time. However, here again, if you find that they are not for you then stop doing them. No one knows your own body better than you. Be aware of this, and you will be able to trust your own judgement.

One thing that is vital is to cleanse the skin properly, to get rid of excess oil, perspiration, air pollutants and dead cells that accumulate on the skin's surface.

In spite of the wide range of cleansers available, soap is still the most common substance used for this. If you use soap and you find that your skin looks and feels good, then soap is right for you. If your skin feels too 'dried out' after washing with soap and water, though, then perhaps you should try a soap with different ingredients, or one of the many facial washes on the market.

When using soap or a facial wash, always wet the skin first. Then make a good lather in your hands before applying it to the face.

Rinsing is very important. You should rinse your face with plenty of warm water – at least twenty splashes. Finish off with a splash of cold water – unless you tend to develop those tiny red veins, in which case it is better to finish with only tepid water.

Never just leave the skin to dry by itself – always dry it thoroughly, ideally with a soft towel. Even if using a facial water spray, always dry your face afterwards, even if only by patting dry with a tissue.

Soaps do not suit everyone, though, and a good alternative is to use a cream or a milky cleanser.

With some cleansers, it is suggested that you follow them with some form of astringent, tonic or skin-freshener, to remove the layer of grease left by the cleanser. The problem is that these also remove some of the skin's natural oils at the same time, so it is inadvisable to use these even only occasionally. It could certainly be extremely harmful to use them daily over a long period, as, whatever your skin type, this could eventually lead to a 'dried-out' skin. A safer alternative is to use a water-soluble cleanser that can be washed/rinsed off after use.

If you use make-up, then I think it is essential to use a creamy cleanser, applying the cleanser to the face and removing with cotton wool or a tissue. This procedure needs to be continued until every trace of 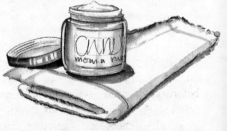 make-up has been removed. Follow this with a light wash, then plenty of water splashes before drying thoroughly. This is my preferred regime.

When you are cleansing your skin, you should be careful that you are removing the dirt and *not* rubbing it in. Gentle, upward, circular strokes are best, to avoid the possibility of the skin being dragged downwards.

To remove eye make-up, I recommend Vaseline. This not only removes the eye make-up but also acts as an excellent lubricant for the delicate skin around the eyes. I find this much better than using eye creams or gels.

Once a week it is a good idea to use some form of preparation to remove any dead cells on the surface of the skin that have not been removed by your daily cleansing routine. The products that do this are called exfoliants, and they usually consist of tiny grains in a cream or gel base. Applied to the face with gentle friction and then rinsed off according to the maker's instructions, they can leave the skin with a fresher and brighter look.

As an alternative to using commercial exfoliants, wet your face with water, then lather your hands with a facial wash, soap or whatever and add a level teaspoon of salt to the lather. Lather your hands again and then wash your face, with light friction. Rinse off well with water, and dry your skin thoroughly.

You should be very careful when you first start to use any exfoliant method. Work very lightly, so as not to damage or irritate the skin's surface. The skin may become less sensitive in time, but don't overdo the treatment to begin with.

A brisk rub over with a soft towel is another excellent way to remove dead cells. It is best done in the morning, before you touch your face with water or anything else. Just rub the towel over your face for about a minute. This is wonderful for the circulation, too – it really feels good. You can use this technique to boost your circulation at other times, but as an exfoliant it will work best first thing in the morning, when you get up.

Face masks are excellent for ridding the skin of impurities and for a smoother face. There are many types on the market. Some come in the form of a cream which dries to a mask when applied to the face. After ten minutes or so the mask is washed off, leaving the skin looking firmer and brighter. Others come in gel form, and, as they usually don't dry or tighten on the face, these may be better for more lined or wrinkled skin.

What should you use on your skin at night? In my opinion, nothing at all! Or, rather, nothing as a general rule. Some form of night cream *is* necessary on occasions – when your skin feels taut, or if the weather is particularly cold.

Oily preparations used on the face to prevent dryness can very often have the opposite effect – clogging the pores and making the skin look slack and dull, while leaving it unable to restore its own natural lubricants. (This applies to oils from vitamin capsules and baby oils, among others.)

Similarly, the regular use of astringent-type preparations to try to improve oily skin *can* worsen that condition too. If that is not your experience, then you have obviously chosen what's right for you; otherwise, try using preparations that are for a so-called 'normal' skin or 'combination' skin (though, here again, veer towards those with a less oily content).

Some creams and, in particular, oils seem to have a very slackening effect on the facial contour. Watch out for this, and try something else if you notice it happening.

As in most things, finding what suits you best all comes down to trial and error. *Don't* use a particular product just because someone else thinks it is good. Occasionally someone will tell me with pride that she has used a particular preparation for years, as did her mother before her. In

nearly every case, the result is not good. You really do
have to find out what is best for *you*.

If your skin feels 'dried out', check your cleansing routine. Are you using a skin toner? If so, perhaps this is
causing dryness. Or it may be that you are suffering from a
vitamin deficiency (see page 156). Night creams – used
sparingly – can definitely benefit the skin at times of stress,
but I do think they are quite ageing if used regularly.

As to moisturizers, I feel that these are fine if used under
some other product. For example, you might use a moisturizer sparingly under your make-up – but *never* apply a
moisturizer to the skin surrounding the eyes. Many moistur-
izing creams work by drawing moisture to the surface of
the skin from the tissue beneath. This may give your
surface skin a more youthful appearance at the expense of
drying out the layers beneath. If you wear some other
product over these creams, as suggested, the evaporation
from the surface isn't so great.

Wearing make-up during the day can provide excellent
protection for the skin. Wind, rain, heat, cold and pollution
can be very harsh, but make-up of some kind can be a
great buffer against these.

There are now make-ups on the market that are so
natural-looking that they are almost undetectable. 'So why
use them?' you might ask. The answer: for protection! And
they do add 'something' to the complexion, however
subtle.

Make-up – whether heavy, light or non-existent – is a
matter of personal choice. You should use whatever makes
you happy and more confident (though skins that are very
lined or wrinkled usually look better with only very light
make-up, with not too much powder).

On the following pages you will find some facial toning
exercises which have a very stimulating effect.

I am very much against the usual facial massage with

creams or oils. Massage is excellent for the body, where the skin can move easily in relation to the muscles beneath. But the skin on the face is directly attached to the under-lying structure, and the link should not be disturbed.

The facial toning methods described here can be practised at any time. Before you begin, though, it is a good idea to

- put yourself in a state of relaxation;
- let yourself go, physically and mentally;
- close your eyes and imagine yourself at a time when you feel completely at one with yourself – really picture this scene;
- breathe naturally and calmly.

When you are ready, open your eyes and proceed.

This relaxation technique can be carried out anywhere, any time. Try it now – it is a very uplifting experience.

TONING AND STIMULATING ROUTINES

You should always carry out these routines with a clean skin.
See the previous section for advice on skin cleansing.

Before you start these routines:

1 Place the palms of your hands together, fingers facing upwards.

2 Now rub the palms of your hands and your wrists together briskly for at least ten seconds.

3 Continue at once with the following toning routines.

The following four toning routines should be carried out in a continuous motion, keeping your hands constantly in touch with your face.

You will obviously have to study the routines before you can do this. Then it is very simple.

TONING ROUTINE 1

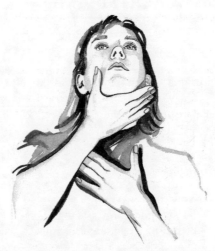

1 Starting with the flat of your *right hand* on your chest, lightly stroke up the front of your neck, under your chin and over your jaw line.

2 Immediately follow with the flat of your *left hand* on your chest, again smoothing upwards and over your neck and your jaw line.

3 Continue alternating your hands like this for at least ten strokes with each hand.

Then, without lifting your hands from your face, continue with the next routine.

TONING ROUTINE 2

With a *featherlight* touch, smooth the palms and fingers of your hands over your face:

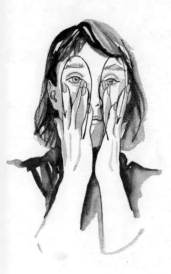

1 Start at your jaw line.

2 Move up and over your cheeks and each side of your nostrils.

3 Then continue gently over the eyes.

4 Now move over the forehead to your hairline.

5 And continue back down the sides of your face to the jaw line.

Repeat these light stroking movements five to ten times, in a continuous motion.

Remember, use very light, smooth strokes – do not stretch the skin at all.

Then, without lifting your hands from your face, continue with the next routine.

TONING ROUTINE 3

1 Glide your middle fingers up towards the bridge of your nose.

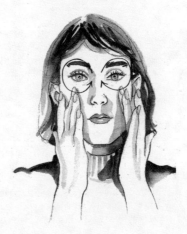

2 Now make circular movements around your eyes.

3 Move from the bridge of your nose along your eyebrows.

4 Now continue down on to your cheekbones and in towards the bridge of your nose again.

Make ten of these light, circular movements.

Then, without lifting your hands from your face, continue with the next routine.

TONING ROUTINE 4

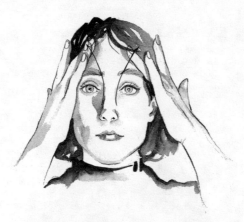

1 With your middle fingers on the bridge
   of your nose, continue upwards
   towards your forehead.

2 With several fingers on your forehead,
   smooth outwards towards your
   temples and hold for a moment with a
   slight pressure.

3 Then continue lightly down each side of
   your face towards your cheekbones in
   a circular movement, coming in
   towards the bridge of your nose.

Repeat this sequence ten times.

*All four toning routines should be carried out in a continuous
motion, without lifting your hands from your face.*

TO INCREASE CIRCULATION IN THE FACE

With the pads of your middle fingers, tap twenty times at the position of each of the dots shown in the illustration below. Make sharp, light, *very quick* taps – like testing a very hot iron.

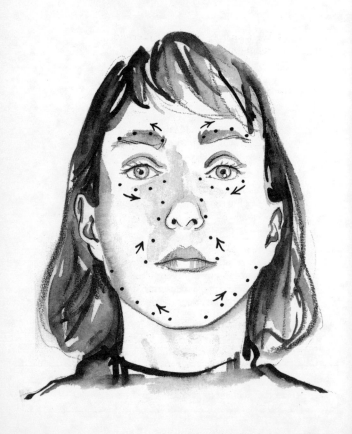

TO INCREASE CIRCULATION IN THE FACE

1 Start on your eyebrows, near the bridge of your nose.
   Tap twenty times at each point.

2 Then make twenty taps on your cheekbones (*not* in your eye sockets).

3 Work up from your mouth corners, ending each side of your nostrils.

4 Work outwards from the centre of your chin, finishing near your ear lobes – tap *not on the jaw bone* but slightly above, on the fleshy area.

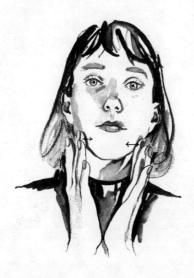

EAR MASSAGE

This massage is very warming and stimulating. Try it – your face will glow!

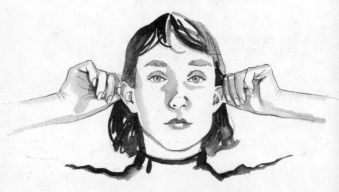

1 With your index fingers and thumbs, hold the top rim of your ears and pull upwards. With small rotations between fingers and thumbs, massage this area.

2 Move down around the rim of the ears, pulling the ears out gently and massaging. Continue like this all around the rim of the ears.

3 When you reach the lobes, pull the lobes down slightly and massage them for about one minute.

Repeat this sequence.

Then, using small, quick, circular movements, massage all the crevices or spirals of the ears. It is best to use the surface of the nails of your index fingers for this; alternatively, you can use the pads of your middle fingers.

TO STIMULATE THE UNDER-CHIN AREA

Slap under your chin with the back of one hand – about thirty quick, light slaps.

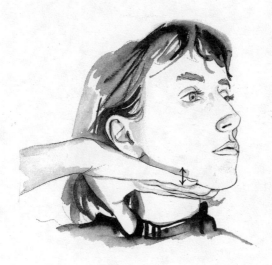

TO STIMULATE HAIR GROWTH

With the pads of your fingertips, massage all over your scalp with small rotations on each point. Do this for at least thirty seconds.

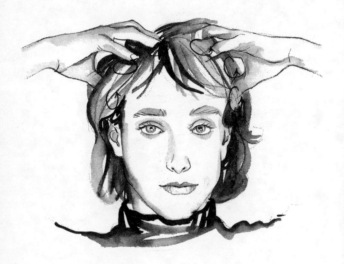

Take large fistfuls of hair and pull upwards.

Clench your hands and lightly pound your scalp with your fists – twenty times.

TO STIMULATE THE LYMPH NODES

Massaging under the jaw bone will stimulate the lymph nodes,
which in turn will help to improve the skin texture.

Hook your thumbs under your jaw
bone, as shown in the illustration. Then
massage deeply, making circular
rotations.

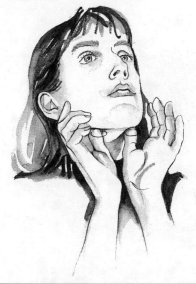

*Start at the outer jaw and work towards the
centre, under your chin.*

This exercise may be painful at first; however, this is quite usual.
After a few days this discomfort will lessen, and eventually this
exercise will be pain-free.

THROAT MASSAGE

This routine is another beautifier for the skin.

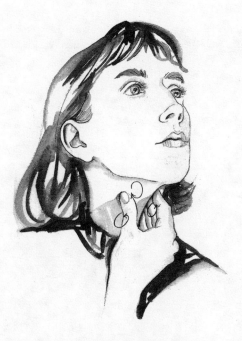

Position the fingers of one hand on one side of your throat and the thumb on the other, as shown in the illustration.

Make rapid circular rotations up and down your throat.

Repeat this with the other hand.

TO STIMULATE THE GUMS

With your fingertips or knuckles, make
circular rotations just above the jaw line,
as shown in the illustration.

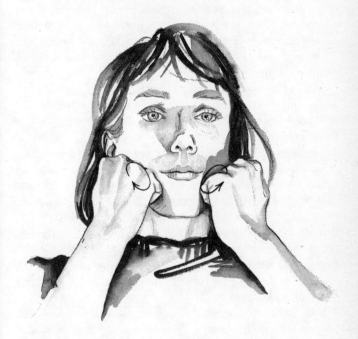

COSMETICS

Many people wrote to me to say how much they enjoyed the section on make-up in my last book. However, some felt that they would have liked to know more – in particular about how to apply make-up to suit different eye shapes, lip shapes and so on. Certainly many people seem to have problems with applying eye shadow.

Ideas about make-up have changed enormously over the years, but many of us are still using the same techniques that we learned in our youth, which often means applying far too much colour.

Fashions in everything change with time, and make-up is no exception. However, I find that I am often slower to take up a new look than many other people – having thick eyebrows when it has become fashionable to have almost none, for example, then starting to pluck them just before heavy brows come in again. This doesn't bother me, though – I prefer to choose whatever I feel suits me best at the time. However, there are some fashions which do definitely go right out, and it is these that need to be reconsidered every now and then.

Over the last few years, the use of eye shadow has probably changed more than any other aspect of make-up, and is probably the most difficult technique to get right.

This all ties in with a chance meeting I had with Christina Stewart of Cosmetics à la Carte in London. Christina is not only a very gifted make-up artist but is also a chemist who manufactures her own range of cosmetics – none of which is tested on animals, I was delighted to find. Her ideas on make-up application were fairly akin to my own, so I was very pleased to discuss her techniques with her, and to pass them on to you.

In the section on skin care, I have already mentioned my belief in wearing some form of protection for the facial skin during the day. This is really necessary all the year round: against the cold and harsh winds in winter, against the harmful rays of the sun in summer, and against pollution in the atmosphere whatever the season.

Fortunately, modern skin-care products are so light that many of them are almost undetectable on the skin. This means that even those of you who don't like the look of any style of make-up can still protect your skins with these new products if you wish. The ideal make-up is no longer heavy-looking. Cosmetics are now very light in texture, and they are long-lasting if they are applied correctly, as you will see.

Always use a mirror in a good light when you are applying make-up – preferably daylight if your make-up is for daytime, but artificial light if it is for after dark.

Before you start applying make-up, it is important to remove every trace of stale make-up, dirt and grease. It is equally important to cleanse the skin in the morning and at night. Overnight, a considerable amount of activity takes place in the body while we sleep. The skin sheds dead cells and secretes sweat and sebum while the body is warm and at rest.

If the skin is prepared carefully and you start the day clean and cool, your make-up will look good for longer. Ideally, it should last until it's time to remove it.

As I said earlier, when you are cleansing your skin, you should be careful that you are removing the dirt and *not* rubbing it in. Gentle, upward, circular strokes are best, to avoid the possibility of the skin being dragged downwards.

Now, with the skin thoroughly clean, a light, greaseless moisturizer can be applied to the face and neck. I differ from some people in that I would *never* put any moisturizer around the eye area, as I explained in the section on skin care.

Next the foundation should be applied. Each of us has a completely unique skin colouring, so it is important to find the right shade of foundation for you. In most cases this will be a shade which tones in with the skin on your cheek just above your jaw line. Test this out at a cosmetics counter when you next need a foundation – the consultant will be happy to help. To get this right, you need to check in daylight, though.

Cosmetics à la Carte specializes in blending its own foundations to match your skin tone exactly. Unfortunately, however, they are not established in every part of the country at present. (Phone the number in the list of useful contacts and addresses at the end of the book to find the nearest centre to you at the moment.)

Having chosen the correct shade of foundation – one that blends exactly with your skin, so that you don't have a mask-like appearance – you then have to apply it properly to achieve a lasting and natural look.

Place *small* dots of foundation on the face and spread it evenly over the skin with a cosmetics sponge. Christina Stewart always advises the use of a sponge, as this avoids the possibility of rubbing the product *into* the skin, like an ointment.

Always apply foundation with light, downward movements. The face is covered with very fine hairs for protection, like a peach, and smoothing the sponge gently downwards in the direction of growth of these little hairs ensures that a fine film of colour is applied, which gives a smoother appearance. Any excess foundation is removed by using the same light smoothing process with a clean part of the sponge.

Using a cosmetics sponge can be quite tricky at first, until you get used to it. Do try it, though, and see how you get on. If you find that you don't like using a sponge, though, apply your foundation in the same way – with light, downward strokes – but using your fingertips instead.

The fine layer of colour applied like this, whether with a sponge or your fingertips, will last all day or all evening, until it is removed with a cleansing lotion or cream. Remember: the less foundation you use, the longer your make-up will last. Some women say that their make-up fades after only a few hours – this usually means that they are using *too much* foundation.

There are several different types of foundation. The 'all-in-one' bases which incorporate face powder are generally popular because they are quicker to use; however, they do have to be retouched quite often.

There are also light products based on moisturizer formulae, with sunscreens added as well as colour. These give a slightly shiny look which can be very attractive, particularly in the summer months.

My favourites – by a long way – are the water-based foundations. These are suitable for all skin types at any age, whereas some of the oil-based products have a definite ageing effect on the skin and you would need to work overtime on your facial exercises to try to counteract this.

Correctly applied, foundation can overcome many defects on the skin's surface – such as shadows, red veins, scars and general blotchiness. If some areas still seem to need extra colour after the application of the base, however, there are concealant products which, applied lightly after the foundation, will blot out any remaining blemishes. Concealer should be applied with a small brush and should *not* be rubbed in.

Many women are concerned about dark shadows around their eyes. This problem is caused by the heavy blood supply to these most important organs: it is the vein near the surface that causes a blue-tone shadow near the corner of the eye, by the nose. A concealer can be used to disguise this problem too.

There are many theories as to why this condition occurs. A lack of protein in the diet is one theory; lack of exercise is another. For some people these shadows seem to be a natural state, no matter what is tried to counteract them and the use of a concealer that tones in with the make-up base, or a shade lighter, is the best answer.

All the colour used so far has been directly related to the basic skin tone and has aimed to produce an even, flattering finish to the skin. Scars, blemishes and unwanted features have been minimized, but at this stage the overall effect may look somewhat flat. The next step is to apply some colour to the cheeks.

Many women claim that they have no cheekbones, or claim not to know where they are. Of course we all have them, and I must mention here that keeping up with your facial exercises will make an amazing difference to the muscle tone in the upper cheek area, giving the appearance of a good cheekbone structure.

Before you start applying colour, use the fingertips lightly to tap out the position of the cheekbones. Smiling broadly into a mirror is helpful, as it emphasizes the 'bunches' over the cheekbones. This makes sure that the colour is applied upwards, giving a cheerful, lively appearance.

There are two types of cheek colour: cream rouge and powder rouge (blusher).

Cream rouge is always applied immediately after the foundation and then powdered over with a translucent face powder. With a powder rouge, or blusher, you apply the translucent powder after the foundation and the blusher last.

The aim of a blusher is to give a *natural*, healthy glow to the face, so don't use too much of it. You will probably find it better to use a larger brush than the one usually provided in the compact, and it is worth investing in one of these.

Face powder can be regarded solely as a setting agent. The modern translucent powders are very fine, and only a little should be pressed well into the make-up and concealer. This gives the translucent effect and results in a truly long-lasting make-up.

Finish by brushing off any excess powder with a large complexion brush. This is a larger brush than the one used for your blusher and is another worthwhile investment.

Now we are ready to move on to the eyes.

The eyes are a most important part of any make-up, but they are a most delicate area and so all heavy, overpowering techniques and products should be avoided. Shiny and pearlized eye-shadows are gradually being superseded by matt products in a variety of pale, muted and sludgy shades. False eyelashes and heavy eye-liners are mainly used for theatrical or special occasions only.

It is now usual to use subtle colours that contrast with the colour of the iris, rather than echoing it. The edges of the various tones are then blended to give a gentle, harmonious effect that will make other people think 'What lovely eyes,' *not* 'What lovely eye make-up.'

It is essential to use the right tools. Brushes are best, and their production need not have been environmentally damaging or unkind to animals: there are excellent synthetic brushes available at a very reasonable cost. Cotton buds are also useful for blending and for removing any excess make-up.

While you are applying the make-up, always keep in mind the final effect that you are aiming to achieve – what clothes you will be wearing, both in style and colour, for example.

A good way to start your eye make-up is to cover virtually the whole eyelid and up to the brow bone with a light matt shadow base, the same shade as the face powder. This will eliminate any further shadows and open the eye area right up.

Always remember that darker shades make things recede; lighter shades bring them forward. Highlights and shadow have complementary effects. Colour is only applied to the face as a highlight when there is bone to support it.

As you will see from the illustrations, different eye shapes need different techniques of eye-shadow application to bring out their full potential.

It is best not to overpluck the eyebrows. If they grow too far down over the brow bone or are extremely untidy, then remove a few stragglers; otherwise the brows look good when they are left quite natural and simply brushed into shape. If they are very light in colour, then a slightly darker shade of eye-shadow can be brushed through them. If they are very thin or stop short, then a few light strokes of a matching shade of eye-pencil can be used, being brushed well to eliminate any hard lines.

The brows and lashes are the natural frame for the eyes. It is a mistake to make them look too hard.

Several thin coats of mascara are preferable to one thick coat. If using an eye-liner, simply place dots in the base of the lower lashes, rather than a solid line.

Kohl pencils should be certificated for use in eye make-up. The use of a kohl line flatters the whites of the eyes, especially in the evening light. A neutral grey or brown can look good with light eyes; black is lovely for really dark eyes.

The face is too small an area to have more than one emphatic feature. So, if the eyes are very dramatic, then the lips should be kept soft and dewy. Conversely, a mouth which is very dramatic in shape and colour needs to be balanced by a muted eye make-up.

Professional make-up artists often use a fine brush to

outline the lips, but using a lip-liner pencil, which tones with the lipstick, is a good and possibly easier way to do this. Using this method, the outline can be improved to some extent. Also, if you have the problem of fine lines round the lips, the pencil line prevents the lipstick running into these. The line should always be gently blended into the lipstick when applied, to prevent a hard line.

After the first application of lipstick, the lips should be blotted gently with a tissue. Face powder is then pressed well into the remaining colour to form an excellent base on to which further lipstick may be applied.

The lasting power of a lipstick depends on the colour content as well as the texture. The glossier the product, the higher the oil content and therefore the easier it is to remove. Matt lipsticks are now becoming available. These are surprisingly light and comfortable to wear, as well as being durable.

For a very natural effect, a lip pencil can be blended over the whole lip area. A touch of lip gloss will make the effect a little more lively.

A narrow upper lip can be emphasized by using a lighter colour, with a slightly darker tone on the lower lip. To achieve an ideal match – perhaps for a dress – you may have to use more than one colour.

There are no hard and fast rules – colour is usually chosen to harmonize with whatever you are wearing. It is a good idea to have several lipsticks, so that you can mix and match to suit both your mood and the circumstances.

The art of all good make-up is to emphasize the good features – and we *all* have them.

Some points to remember:
● Less foundation is better than more.
● Water-based foundations are excellent for any skin type and any age.

- Blusher should be used sparingly – its purpose is to give you a natural healthy glow.
- Most importantly: if you can't get a perfect result, remember that make-up is only fun anyway.

Eye-shadows should basically be muted neutral shades. Never use shades that overpower your own eye colour, such as bright blues or greens.

Get advice if you are not sure about colour and application. Even with advice, you will probably have to experiment. It is essential to do this in a good light.

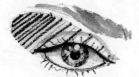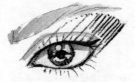

CLOSE-SET EYE – BROWS LOW SET

Begin with the lightest shades at the inner corners of the eyes, blending upwards and outwards to the corners with a darker shade.

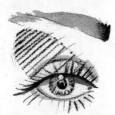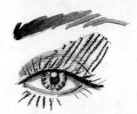

HOODED EYES THAT DROOP AT THE OUTER CORNERS

Stop your eye-shadow before you reach the outer corners of your eyes. Use mascara to emphasize the lashes at the centre of the eyes.

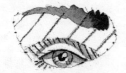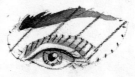

SMALL EYES

To make small eyes look bigger, cover the whole of the lid up to the brow with a light shadow as a foundation. Contour the crease with a muted shade and blend in.

The shape of your lips can be very slightly improved.

It is easier to make the new outline with a lip-liner pencil and then fill in with a lipstick applied with a lip brush.

Lightly blot your lipstick, apply a little powder and blot again. Then apply a second coat of lipstick.

FOR LIPS THAT ARE TOO FULL

With a lip-liner pencil, draw just inside your own natural lip line but take this line well out to the corners.

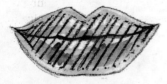

Fill in this area with lipstick – not glossy.

FOR DROOPY MOUTH CORNERS

With a lip-liner pencil, extend your lower lip slightly upwards at the corners.

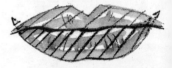

Fill in this area with lipstick applied with a brush. Use a slightly lighter lip colour on the top lip.

FOR THIN LIPS

With a lip-liner pencil, outline the contour of the lips just slightly beyond the natural line.

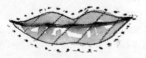

Fill in this area with a lighter lipstick shade.

FOR A THIN TOP LIP

With a lip-liner pencil, draw just inside your lower lip line. Fill in this area with lipstick.

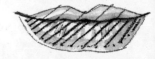

Apply a slightly lighter lipstick to your upper lip.

THE BODY EXERCISE
PROGRAMME

There is no doubt about it: if you keep your body in good working order you will feel less tired, you will be more positive in your outlook and you will be able to accomplish more in your daily activities. You will possibly also sleep more soundly. You will certainly become stronger and more flexible. You will look and feel younger.

However, you need to be sensible when exercising. If you have not been very active, then you should start with a very light routine, gradually adding more to your programme each week. One of the reasons why people give up their exercise routines is because they have tried to do too much at the start and have launched into it so enthusiastically that they have finished up exhausted. It can take weeks to recover from such onslaughts on the body. Unless you are a professional athlete, a workout three or four times a week, with half an hour or so of aerobic activity, should keep you in excellent shape.

There are now so many workout programmes available that it is difficult to know which ones to choose. I have investigated several of the methods available and have tried many of them. While doing this, some time ago, I came across Liz Roberts, who is a qualified personal-fitness trainer. I totally agreed with – and enjoyed – Liz's approach to physical fitness, so between us we have worked out an exercise plan which we hope you will enjoy too. It is safe and suitable for anyone, at any age.

This programme will give you a thorough workout for every part of the body, from head to toe, gently moving all the joints, exercising the muscles and ending each section with a very necessary stretch of the muscles that have just been worked on, to prevent the aches and pains that so many people experience after working out. The warm-up section may seem lengthy, but it isn't really. It is a marvellous routine which should be learned so that you can complete the whole sequence without a break.

The body exercises will work out every part of you – your neck, shoulders and all parts of your arms; your torso; the front, back and sides of your legs; your ankles and toes – ending with a complete relaxation sequence for body and mind. (The face, of course, is well taken care of in the Facial Workout section.)

To complete your fitness programme you will need to take up some kind of aerobic exercise. This is not as difficult as it might seem: it need not involve vigorous activity at the local gym. Any physical exercise that increases the activity of the heart and lungs can be classed as aerobic exercise, so brisk walking, running, jogging, dancing, cycling, swimming and skipping are all suitable.

To be of use, any aerobic activity has to be continuous for *at least* twenty minutes, three or four times a week. Walking needs to be brisk to be really effective, and walking uphill for part of the way, however slight the incline, is more advantageous. Jogging is suitable but not if you have pelvic problems. Even wearing special footwear, the pounding of jogging on hard surfaces such as pavements can put enormous strain on the knees and the lower back. For swimming to have an effect, you would need to swim continuously for thirty minutes.

IMPORTANT

Never attempt a new exercise programme without checking with your doctor that it is safe – particularly if you suffer from heart disease, high blood-pressure, varicose veins or asthma, or if you are overweight or pregnant.

PREPARATION

Preparation is minimal for the following exercise programme.

You will need to wear something unrestrictive, and comfortable – a light-weight tracksuit, a leotard, or tights and a T-shirt are all excellent.

Find a space where you don't feel restricted in your movements. The floor shouldn't be too hard. A carpet, a rug or a folded blanket for the floor work is essential.

You should feel comfortably warm.

It is always easier to work out to music, as it keeps you moving more rhythmically. However, you will need to follow the programme first, to find out the right tempo for you.

Feel at one with yourself before you start. Choose a time when you know you won't be disturbed, and have fun.

WARM-UP EXERCISES

The following warm-up routine is intended to move all your joints systematically. This is essential before any fitness workout. Once you have learned this routine, it is amazingly quick to do and very effective.

Each section of this exercise programme concentrates on a different part of you in turn. For instance, the leg exercises work the back of the leg, then the front, then the sides, and so on.

Try steadily to learn this whole routine – it has an amazing effect. I am sure it will help you as much as it has helped me.

WARM-UP EXERCISE 1

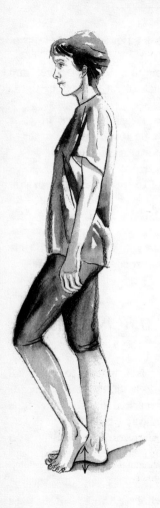

Stand with your feet almost together, your arms down at your sides.

Bend your right knee as you raise and lower your right heel – eight times.

Repeat with your left leg – eight times.

Pause.

Raise and lower your right and left heels alternately – eight times.

WARM-UP EXERCISE 1

Throughout the following three exercises, keep raising and lowering your heels continuously – left, right, left, right.

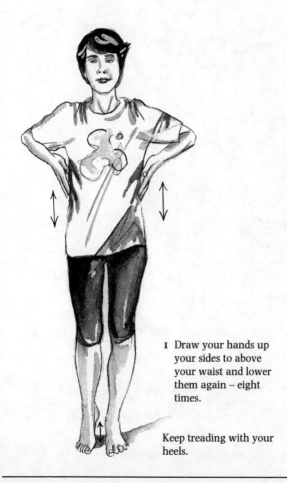

1 Draw your hands up your sides to above your waist and lower them again – eight times.

Keep treading with your heels.

WARM-UP EXERCISE 1

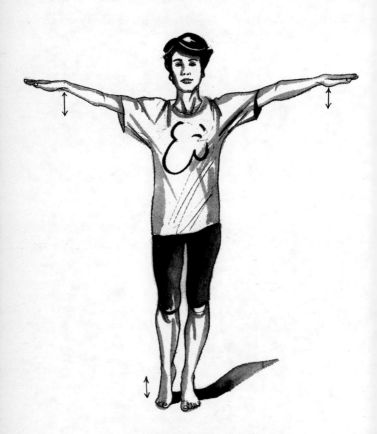

2 Raise your arms from your sides
  straight out to shoulder level and
  lower them again – eight times.

Keep treading with your heels.

WARM-UP EXERCISE 1

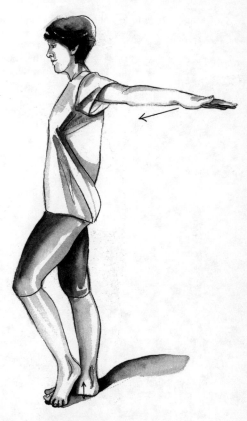

3 Raise your arms straight out to
   shoulder level then push them back
   towards your shoulder-blades – eight
   times.

Now relax.

WARM-UP EXERCISE 2

Stand with your feet at hip distance apart, with your toes
facing forward.

Keep your arms at your side, your tummy in, your bottom under and
your shoulders relaxed throughout.

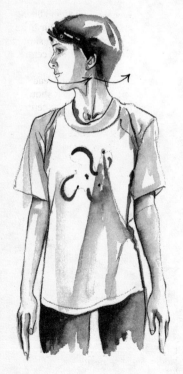

1 Turn your head slowly to the
right, then back to the
centre.

2 Now turn your head slowly
to the left, then back to the
centre.

Do these two movements in a
continuous sequence – eight
times.

WARM-UP EXERCISE 3

Stand with your feet at hip distance apart, with your toes facing forward.

Keep your arms at your side, your tummy in, your bottom under and your shoulders relaxed throughout.

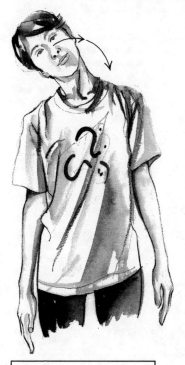

1 Keeping your head facing forward, lower your head towards your right shoulder, then return to the centre.

2 Now lower your head towards your left shoulder, then return to the centre.

Do these two movements in a continuous sequence – eight times.

Do not strain your head down towards your shoulder.

WARM-UP EXERCISE 4

Stand with your feet at hip distance apart, with your toes
facing forward.

Keep your arms at your side, your tummy in, your bottom under and
your shoulders relaxed throughout.

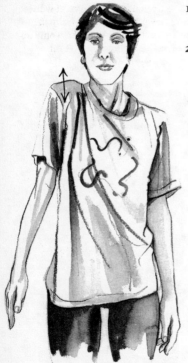

1 Lift your left shoulder up and
down – four times.

2 Lift your right shoulder up
and down – four times.

WARM-UP EXERCISE 5

Stand with your feet at hip distance apart, with your toes facing
forward, your arms at your sides.

Keep your tummy in, your bottom under and your shoulders
relaxed throughout.

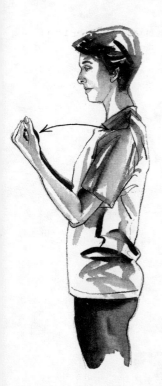

Keeping your elbows at waist
level, bend your arms up in
front so that your fists come up
to your shoulders – eight
times.

WARM-UP EXERCISE 6

Stand with your feet at hip distance apart, with your toes facing forward, your arms at your side.

Keep your tummy in, your bottom under and your shoulders relaxed throughout.

Raise your arms straight out to shoulder level, then swing your forearms up and down from your elbows – eight times.

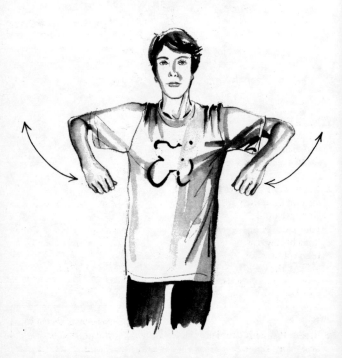

WARM-UP EXERCISE 7

Stand with your feet wide apart, with your legs straight and your toes facing forward, your arms at your side.

Keep your tummy in, your bottom under and your shoulders relaxed throughout.

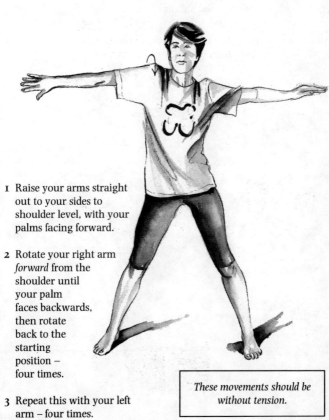

1 Raise your arms straight out to your sides to shoulder level, with your palms facing forward.

2 Rotate your right arm *forward* from the shoulder until your palm faces backwards, then rotate back to the starting position – four times.

3 Repeat this with your left arm – four times.

These movements should be without tension.

95

WARM-UP EXERCISE 8

Stand with your feet wide apart, with your legs straight and your toes facing forward, your arms at your sides.

Keep your tummy in, your bottom under and your shoulders relaxed throughout.

Bend gently sideways from the waist – eight times to the left, then eight times to the right.

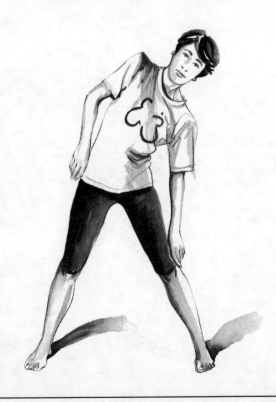

WARM-UP EXERCISE 9

Stand with your feet wide apart, with your knees bent and your toes
pointing outward.

Keep your tummy in, your bottom under and your shoulders
relaxed throughout.

1 Raise your arms out to the sides at
shoulder level, palms facing down.

2 Keeping your body upright, stretch out
your arms and ribs first to one side
and then to the other – eight times.

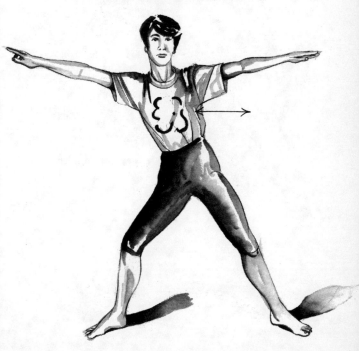

WARM-UP EXERCISE 10

Stand with your feet wide apart, with your legs straight and your toes facing forward.

Keep your arms at your sides, your tummy in, your bottom under and your shoulders relaxed throughout.

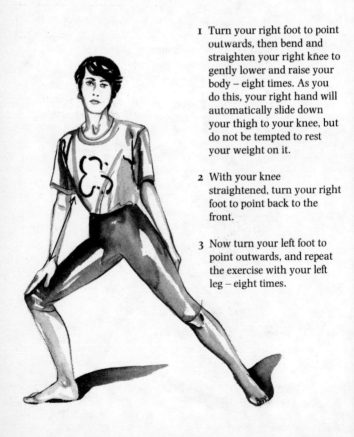

1 Turn your right foot to point outwards, then bend and straighten your right knee to gently lower and raise your body – eight times. As you do this, your right hand will automatically slide down your thigh to your knee, but do not be tempted to rest your weight on it.

2 With your knee straightened, turn your right foot to point back to the front.

3 Now turn your left foot to point outwards, and repeat the exercise with your left leg – eight times.

WARM-UP EXERCISE 11

Stand with your feet a little more than hip distance apart, with your knees slightly bent and your toes pointing slightly outwards.

Keep your tummy in, your bottom under and your shoulders relaxed throughout.

> *Don't arch your back.*

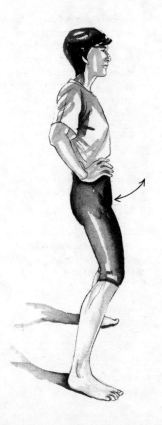

1 With your hands on your hips, tilt your pelvis forward and up, then back to the starting position – eight times.

WARM-UP EXERCISE 11

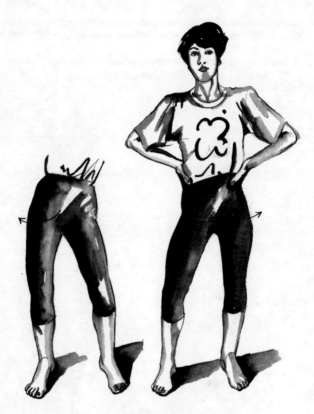

2 Now tilt your pelvis up to the left and back to the starting position – eight times.

3 Then tilt your pelvis up to the right and back to the starting position – eight times.

WARM-UP EXERCISE 12

Stand with your feet together, with your legs straight and your toes facing forward, your hands on your waist.

Keep your arms at your sides, your tummy in, your bottom under and your shoulders relaxed throughout.

1 Lift your right foot forward, just off the floor.

2 Point your foot and bend it back again – eight times.

3 Keeping your foot raised, rotate it outwards – eight times.

4 Now rotate your foot inwards – eight times.

Repeat this sequence with the left foot.

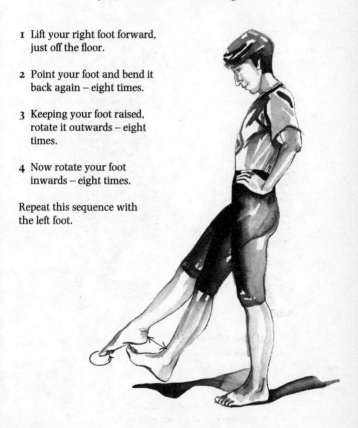

WARM-UP EXERCISE 13

Stand with your feet wide apart, your knees bent and your toes facing outwards, your hands on your waist.

Keep your tummy in, your bottom under and your shoulders relaxed throughout.

1 With the ball of your foot remaining on the floor, lift and lower your right heel – eight times.

2 Repeat with your left heel – eight times.

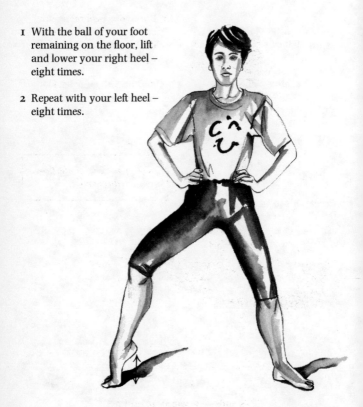

WARM-UP EXERCISE 14

Stand with your feet almost together, your hands on your waist.

Keep your tummy in, your bottom under and your shoulders relaxed throughout.

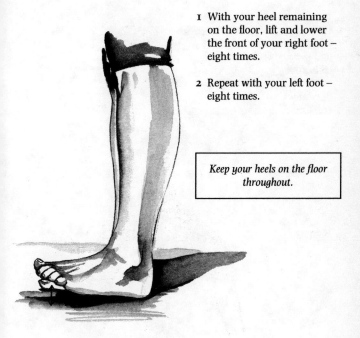

1 With your heel remaining on the floor, lift and lower the front of your right foot – eight times.

2 Repeat with your left foot – eight times.

> *Keep your heels on the floor throughout.*

This ends your warm-up routine.

Now continue immediately with the following arm exercises.

ARM EXERCISES

FOR THE OUTSIDE OF THE UPPER ARMS

Please keep the following continuous foot movement going
throughout the next four exercises.

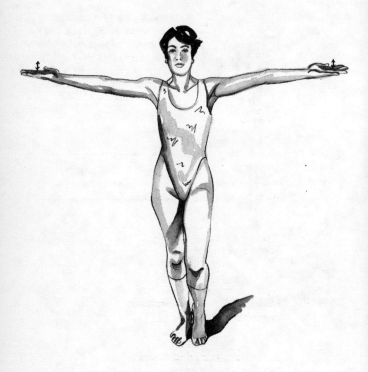

1 Raise your arms from your sides to
shoulder level, with your palms facing
the ceiling.

FOR THE OUTSIDE OF THE UPPER ARMS

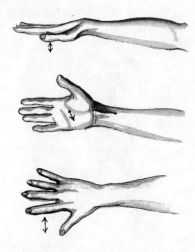

2 With tiny movements, push up and
   down (about 1 inch) – eight times.

3 Repeat with your palms facing
   downwards – eight times.

4 Repeat with your palms facing
   forwards pushing backwards and
   forwards – eight times.

5 Repeat with your palms facing
   backwards – eight times.

Keep your neck relaxed throughout.

FOR THE INSIDE OF THE UPPER ARMS

With your feet together, walk on the spot,
lifting only your heels.

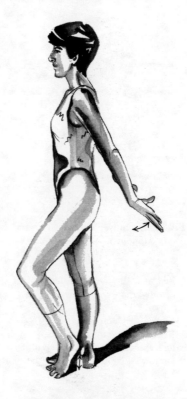

1 With your arms at your sides, palms
facing the back wall and fingers
spread, push your arms straight back
behind you, then make small
additional pushing movements – eight
times.

FOR THE INSIDE OF THE UPPER ARMS

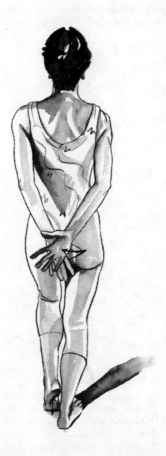

2 Now, keeping your arms in the same
   position, criss-cross your hands behind
   you – eight times.

FOR THE OUTSIDE OF THE LOWER ARMS

With your feet together, walk on the spot, *lifting only your heels.*

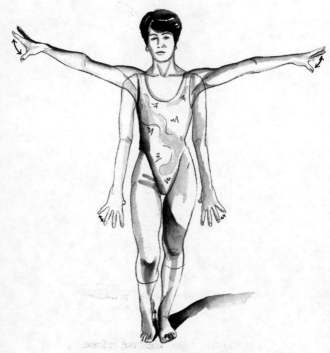

1 With your arms at your sides, clench your fingers then spread them out – eight times.

2 With your arms straight out at shoulder level, clench your fingers then spread them out – eight times.

FOR THE OUTSIDE OF THE LOWER ARMS

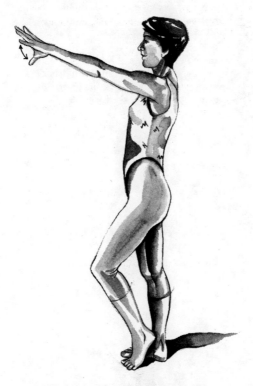

3 With your arms straight out in front,
   clench your fingers then spread them
   out – eight times.

4 Then repeat step 2 – eight times.

5 Then repeat step 1 – eight times.

TO RELAX YOUR ARMS 1

With your feet together, walk on the spot,
lifting only your heels.

Keeping your elbows at waist level,
clench your fists loosely and swing your
arms up to your shoulders and down
again.

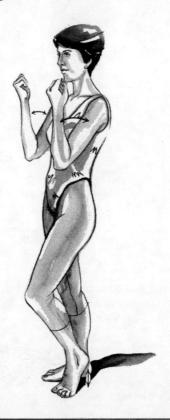

TO RELAX YOUR ARMS 2

With your feet together, walk on the spot,
lifting only your heels.

With your arms out to the sides at
shoulder level, clench your fists loosely
and swing them to the armpits and back,
from the elbows – four times.

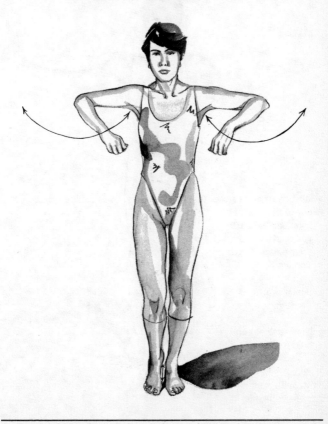

ARMS STRETCH 1

Stand with your feet at hip distance apart.

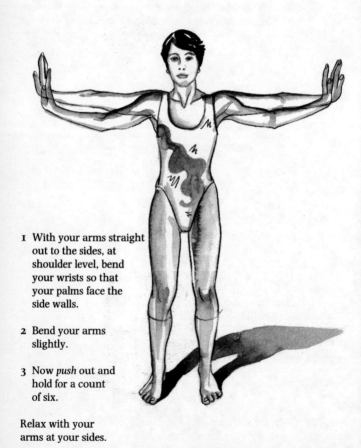

1 With your arms straight
   out to the sides, at
   shoulder level, bend
   your wrists so that
   your palms face the
   side walls.

2 Bend your arms
   slightly.

3 Now *push* out and
   hold for a count
   of six.

Relax with your
arms at your sides.

ARMS STRETCH 2

Stand with your feet at hip distance apart.

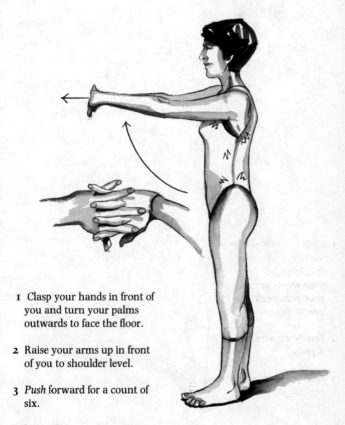

1 Clasp your hands in front of you and turn your palms outwards to face the floor.

2 Raise your arms up in front of you to shoulder level.

3 *Push* forward for a count of six.

Relax with your arms at your sides.

ARMS STRETCH 3

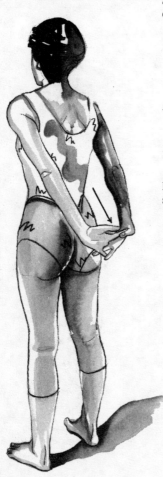

Stand with your feet at hip distance apart.

1 Clasp your hands behind your back and turn your palms outwards to face the floor.

2 Lift your arms as high as you can.

3 Bend your arms and *push* out for a count of six.

Relax with your arms at your sides.

ARMS STRETCH 4

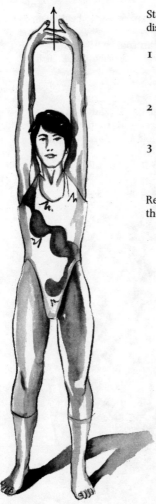

Stand with your feet at hip distance apart.

1 Clasp your hands in front of you with your palms facing downwards.

2 Lift your arms so your palms face the ceiling.

3 Bend your elbows and *push* up with your hands. Hold for a count of six.

Relax your arms and shake them out.

ARMS STRETCH 5

Stand with your knees slightly bent.

1 Stretch up with your right arm then bend your arm at the elbow and reach to touch between your shoulder-blades.

2 With your left hand, gently pull your right elbow over towards the centre of your head. Hold for a count of eight.

3 Now repeat with left arm.

Repeat once more on each side.

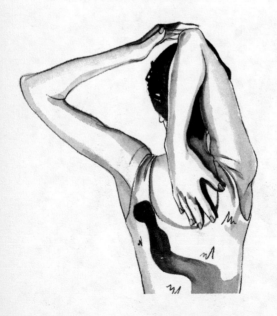

TOTAL BODY STRETCH

Stand with your feet wide apart, your toes pointing outwards.

> *Feel a good stretch at each stage.*

1 Bend your knees as much as possible and at the same time push your outstretched hands down your thighs to your knees.

2 Bring your hands back up, straighten your legs and stretch with your arms above your head.

Do this eight times.

LEG EXERCISES

FOR THE FRONT OF THE THIGHS 1

Lie on the floor with your knees bent.

1 Raise your head off the floor and lightly support it with your hands.

2 Slide your right foot along the floor to straighten the leg.

3 With the foot flexed, lift the straightened leg to the height of the left knee and back down.

Do this eight times.

Then repeat eight times with the toes pointed.

Now repeat this entire exercise with the left leg.

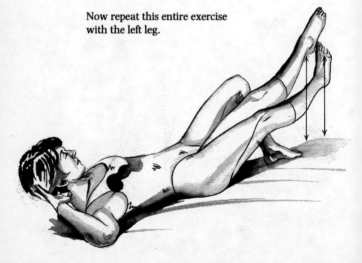

FOR THE FRONT OF THE THIGHS 2

Lie on the floor with your head lightly
supported on your hands.

1 Bend your knees up as shown in the
   diagram.

2 With your feet flexed, straighten your
   legs towards the ceiling, then bend
   them again.

Do this eight times.

Then repeat eight times
with pointed toes.

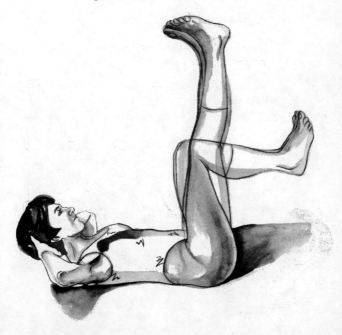

LEGS STRETCH 1

Sit on the floor with your knees bent.

1 Move your right foot sideways and
   back until the heel is level with your
   right hip – at the same time, bend
   your right knee inwards to rest on the
   floor.

2 Lean back on to your forearms, or, if
   this is difficult, on to your hands,
   keeping your knee on the floor. Feel
   the stretch in the front of your leg.

3 Hold for a count of six.

Repeat with the left leg.

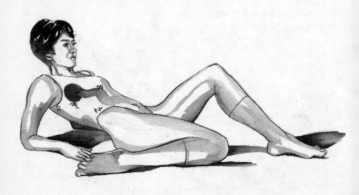

FOR THE SIDE OF THE LEGS

This will exercise the legs at three levels, as shown in the illustration.

Lie on one side, with your head on your hand.
Bend the underneath leg, but keep the
top leg straight.

1 Lift the top leg up to the first level.
Lower slightly and raise to first level again.
Do this eight times.

2 Starting with the top leg at level 1, lift
the leg to level 2 and back to level 1.
Do this eight times.

3 Starting with the top leg at level 2, lift
the leg to level 3 and back to level 2.
Do this eight times.

Now turn over on your other side and repeat the
three stages eight times with your other leg.

*Make sure your elbow, ribs
and hips are in line with
one another and that your
spine is straight.*

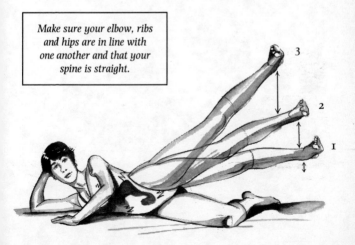

LEGS STRETCH 2

Sit cross-legged on the floor.

1 Place the palms of your hands on the floor in front of your feet.

2 Lower yourself forward on to your forearms. Feel the stretch at the back and side of your legs.

3 Hold for a count of six.

Release and relax.

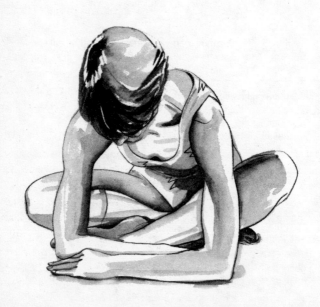

FOR THE BACK OF THE LEGS 1

Lie on one side and take all your upper
body weight on to the lower arms.

1 With your legs straight and your top
   foot flexed, lift your upper leg up and
   backwards as far as possible.

2 Release the tension slightly and lift
   again – eight times.

Repeat on the other side – eight times.

> *Don't forget to breathe.*

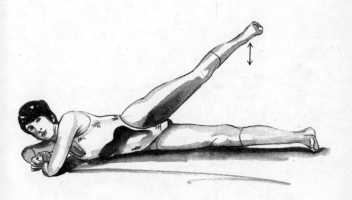

FOR THE BACK OF THE LEGS 2

Start on all fours and then rest on your forearms.

1 With the toes pointed, slide your right foot along the floor behind you to stretch the right leg.

2 Now lift your right leg up as high as you can, cross it over your left leg and lower it to the floor.

3 Lift your right leg up again and back to the resting position.

Do this eight times.

Then repeat with your left leg – eight times.

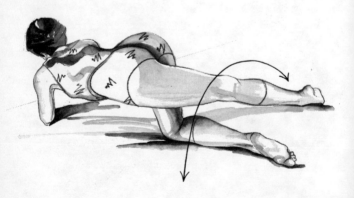

FOR THE BACK OF THE LEGS 3

Start on all fours then rest on your
forearms.

1 Lift your right leg up behind you, bent
at the knee.

2 With the foot flexed, lift your right
heel towards the ceiling. Lift and lower
in a pumping action – eight times.

Repeat with your left leg – eight times.

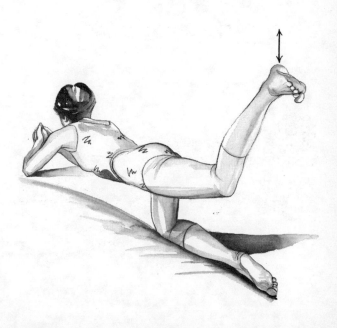

LEGS STRETCH 3

Lie on the floor with your knees bent.

1 Bring your right knee up on to your chest.

2 Hold the right ankle steady with both hands, then ease your right knee in towards your right armpit.

3 Hold for a count of six, then release.

Repeat with the left leg.

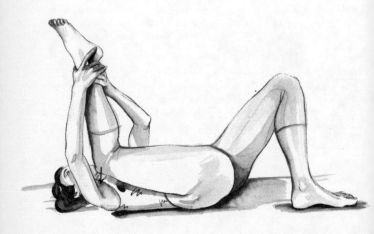

FOR THE INNER THIGH 1

Lie on your right side and rest your head on your hand.

> *Everything must be in line through your shoulder, ribs and hips.*

1 Keeping your right leg straight, bend your left leg and rest your left foot on the floor in front of you.

2 With your right foot flexed, raise and lower your straight right leg without it touching the floor – eight times.

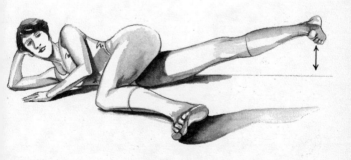

FOR THE INNER THIGH 2

Lie on your right side and rest your head
on your hand.

> *Everything must be in line through your*
> *shoulder, ribs and hips.*

1 Keeping your right leg straight, bend
your left leg and rest your left foot on
the floor in front of you.

2 Place your right forearm on the floor.

3 Pull your left leg up and hold the foot.
Move your right leg slightly forward.

4 Raise and lower the straight right leg
without it touching the floor – eight
times.

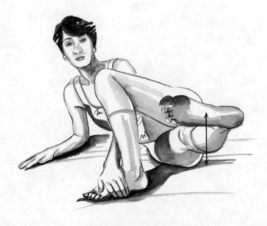

FOR THE INNER THIGH 3

Lie on your right side and rest your head on your hand.

> *Everything must be in line through your shoulder, ribs and hips.*

1 Keeping your right leg straight, bend your left leg and rest your left foot on the floor in front of you.

2 Bring your left knee up towards your chest and rest it on the floor.

3 Bring your right leg further forward, keeping it straight.

4 Raise and lower the straight right leg without it touching the floor – eight times.

Now repeat these last three workouts on the left side.

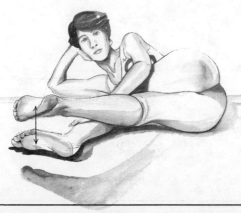

LEGS STRETCH 4

1 Kneel on your left knee with your right
  foot well forward and your toes well
  turned out.

2 Lean forward and rest forearms on
  your right knee.

Hold for a count of six.

Repeat this stretch with the other leg.

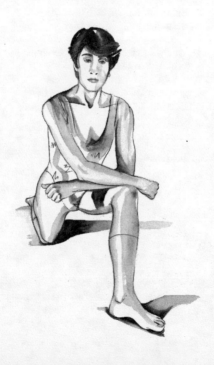

ABDOMINAL EXERCISES

ABDOMINAL EXERCISE 1

Lie on your back with your knees bent.

1 Keeping the balls of your feet on the floor, raise both heels.

2 Lift yourself up on to your forearms – with your palms on the floor.

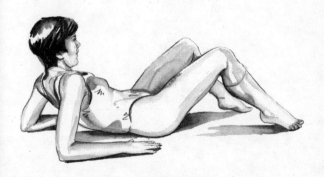

ABDOMINAL EXERCISE 1

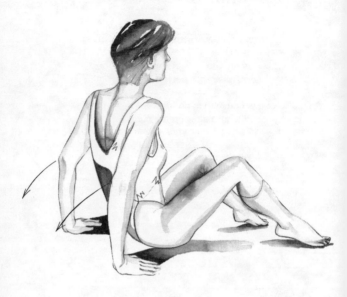

3 Now lift your body to straighten your
   arms.
   Your tummy muscles should be
   working here.

4 Then lean back on to your lower arms
   again.

Do this eight times.

> *Get your tummy muscles working here, not
> your arms.*

ABDOMINAL EXERCISE 2

Lie on your back with your knees bent,
your feet and knees slightly apart.

1 Keeping the balls of your feet on the
floor, lift both heels.

2 Reach forward with your arms and lift
yourself into *almost* a sitting position.
Hold for a count of six.

3 Slowly lower yourself back towards the
floor, keeping your head and shoulders
off the floor.

Lift and lower yourself eight times in all.

Remember to raise your heels off the floor.

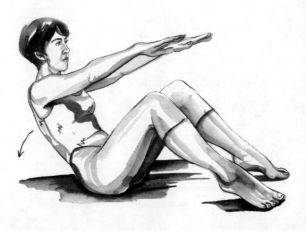

ABDOMINAL EXERCISE 3

Lie on your back with both knees bent
up on to your chest.

1 Lift your head up.

2 Reach forward with your arms
  stretched out on each side of your
  knees.

3 Release slightly, then reach forward
  again – eight times.

*Your head and shoulders should be raised off
the floor throughout this exercise.*

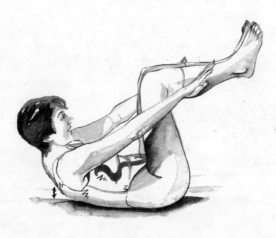

ABDOMINAL EXERCISE 4

Lie on your back with your knees bent.

1 Hold the inside of your thighs, with your hands pushing outwards.

2 Lift yourself into *almost* a sitting position.

3 Lower yourself back, keeping your head and shoulders off the floor.

Slowly lift and lower yourself eight times in all.

> *Feel your tummy muscles working here.*

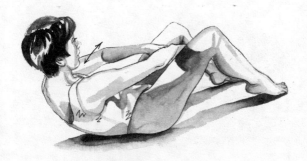

ABDOMINAL EXERCISE 5

Lie on your back.

1 Bend your knees towards your chest
and cross your ankles, spreading your
knees wide apart.

2 With your hands behind your head,
lift your right elbow to your left knee
then lower yourself back to the floor –
eight times.

3 Repeat with the left elbow to the right
knee – eight times.

4 Then repeat with both elbows to both
knees – eight times.

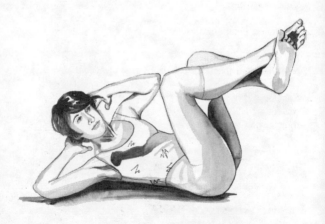

ABDOMINAL EXERCISE 6

Lie on your back. Bring your knees up, as shown in the diagram, and cross your ankles.

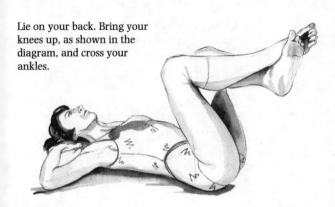

1 Straighten your legs to the ceiling then slightly bend your knees.

2 Raise your head slightly.

3 Lift your arms up and reach for your toes.

4 Release slightly and reach again – eight times in all.

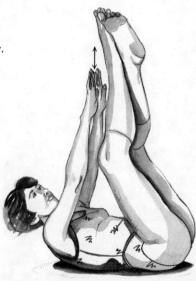

DIAGONAL STRETCH

Lie on the floor with your knees bent, your arms straight out at your sides to form a T-shape.

Breathe in.

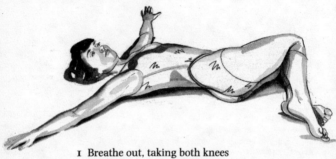

1 Breathe out, taking both knees together over to the left side on to the floor.

2 Breathe in, bringing your knees back to centre.

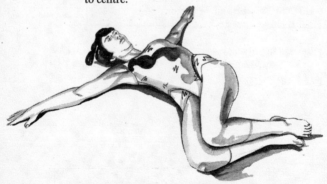

3 Breathe out, taking both knees over to the right side on to the floor.

DIAGONAL STRETCH

4 Breathe in, bringing your knees back
   to the centre.
   Feel the stretch down your back.

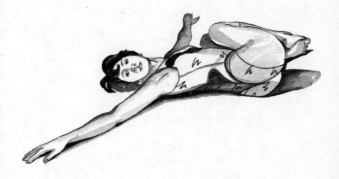

5 Now take both knees over to the left
   side, drawing your knees up towards
   your left arm.

6 Turn your head to the right for a count
   of six.

7 Bring your head back to the centre.

8 Centre your knees.

9 Repeat on other side.

> *Keep your arms and shoulders firmly on the*
> *floor throughout.*

BOTTOM EXERCISES

BOTTOM EXERCISE 1

Lie on the floor with your knees bent,
your feet at hip distance apart.

1 Raise your toes, keeping your *heels on
   the floor*.

2 Raise your head and support it with
   your hands.

3 Lift your bottom off the floor.

4 Tense and release the bottom muscles
   – eight times.

Relax with your bottom, head and toes
back on the floor.

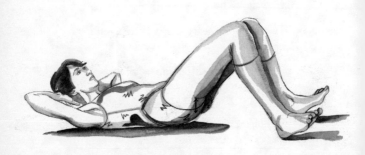

BOTTOM EXERCISE 2

Lie on your back with your knees bent,
your feet and knees together.

1 Push your feet a few inches further
   away from your bottom.

2 Raise your head and support it with
   your hands.

3 Lift your bottom off the floor.

4 Tense and release the bottom muscles
   – eight times.

Relax with your bottom and head back
on the floor.

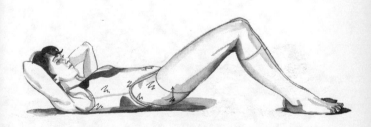

BOTTOM EXERCISE 3

Lie on your back with your knees bent, your feet and knees together.

1 Push your feet a few inches further away from your bottom.

2 Raise your head and support it with your hands.

3 Straighten your right leg and raise it to left-knee level.

4 Lift your bottom off the floor.

5 Tense and release the bottom muscles – eight times.

Repeat with your left leg raised – eight times.

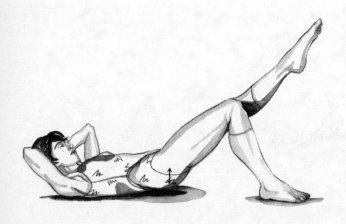

BOTTOM EXERCISE 4

Lie on the floor with your knees bent,
your feet more than hip distance apart.

1 Raise your head and support it with
   your hands.

2 With your knees apart, lift your
   bottom.

3 Tense and release the bottom muscles.

4 Bring your knees together.

5 Tense and release the bottom muscles.

Do this eight times.

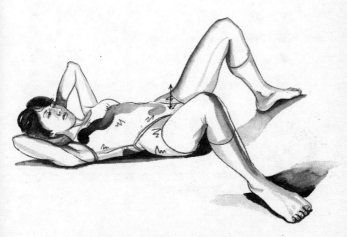

Now repeat the Diagonal Stretch on page 138.

FOR TOTAL RELAXATION

Feel very calm and at peace with yourself throughout

While learning this relaxation technique, it is useful to have someone slowly read the instructions out for you to follow. Alternatively, record the instructions on to a cassette.

Lie flat out on the floor.

Let your feet fall away from each other.

Shake your legs out.

Rest your hands on your hips.

Lift up your head slowly and then lower it back down.

Close your eyes.

Breathe in and out deeply.

Keep your head on the floor, lower your chin towards your chest and release it again.

Push your head into the floor and release it again.

Push your shoulders down and release them again.

Push your elbows out and release them again (still keeping your hands resting on your hips).

Stretch your fingers and thumbs well apart and release them again.

FOR TOTAL RELAXATION

Bring your arms down to your sides, with your palms facing the ceiling.

Push your shoulders down and release them again.

Push your hands and arms into the floor and release them again.

Push your lower back into the floor and relax it again.

Point your toes, stretch your feet and legs, and release them again.

Flex your feet, push your heels away and release them again.

Spread your toes and release them again.

Breathe in and out deeply – ten times.

Gently curl up on to your side.

Roll on to all fours.

Gently push back on to your feet.

Very slowly uncurl into a standing position.

If it makes you more comfortable, place a cushion under your knees.

THE FINAL STRETCH

Stand with your feet wide apart, your toes pointing outwards.

1 Lift your arms straight out, with your wrists crossed in front of you.
  Bend your knees.

2 Now straighten your legs – at the same time swinging your arms out to the sides and recrossing your wrists above your head.

3 Swing down, bending your knees and crossing your wrists in front of you.

Do this three times.

These should be very relaxed free swinging movements.

HEALTH, DIET AND DIETING

Health, diet and dieting must be the most written-about subjects in the world, and possibly the most controversial – which is not surprising, for what suits you could well be not at all suitable for me. It is imperative that each and every one of us learns to become aware of and to understand our own individual needs.

This is not as difficult as it may seem. For example, headaches, aches and pains are signals that all is not well. The symptoms may be quite minor, but nevertheless they should not be ignored. Many people tend to accept these small ailments as inevitable, thinking that everyone has them. This may or may not be so, but in any case you should ask yourself one question: why?

I, for one, would be very unhappy to have a recurring symptom and yet do nothing about it, other than perhaps take a painkiller, until it comes round again. But many people seem to exist in this way.

With a little self-analysis, it is usually possible to work back to an understanding of what has brought about a particular malaise. For example, is tension the problem? If so, what has caused it?

Many headaches can be cured – or, better still, prevented by simply sitting quietly and relaxing your forehead, your eyes and your neck and shoulder muscles. Close your eyes – not tightly, though, as that would create even more tension – and feel calm and at peace. (See page 144).

Headaches and other forms of tension can be caused by the stress of demanding too much of yourself – being too self-critical. If this is the case, stop being so hard on yourself. No one is perfect all the time. If you are doing your best then you have to accept this. When you are sitting quietly relaxed, praise yourself for what you *have* achieved.

You also need to feel confident about your appearance, about yourself. I find that this is a problem for many people – they are critical of their features, their hair, their figures – and this applies to people in all walks of life. Many of these people are in fact extremely attractive – some even beautiful – and yet they have these hang-ups. I can understand this, for we all seem to have similar problems and fears in our lives from time to time. The important thing is to do something about it.

Other aches and pains can be caused by certain foods. Could it be that you are eating or drinking something that doesn't agree with *your* system? Aches and pains of a rheumatic nature can sometimes be caused by particular foods, and – surprisingly – depressions are often caused by foods we eat or by some form of drink.

You need to consider every food category when investigating this. Even a particular fruit could be responsible, for it is not simply the 'bad' foods that can cause adverse symptoms.

And do not overlook the effects that tea and/or coffee can have on your system – they can often lead to nervousness and irritability. Being aware, in this instance, could mean that you no longer have to resort to tranquillizers or harmful medication.

It is important to investigate every avenue that you can think of that might lead to the cause of any recurring dis-ease – it is really worth taking time to do this.

Even if you are used to referring all your aches and pains to your doctor, it is nevertheless helpful if you have made some attempt to trace the cause of the problem yourself.

Doctors obviously don't have time to discuss every patient's life problems – how could they? – so a prescription is all we can expect for most minor ills. I wonder how often a prescription gets to the root of the problem, though. This is not to say that seeking medical advice is pointless – far from it. Some symptoms are a sign of something more serious than we could hope to deal with ourselves. Doctors, hospitals and drugs are all, unfortunately, a necessity for many of us at some times in our lives – and how grateful we are for them in times of need. However, in many ways we are the only ones who can really take care of ourselves – take care, that is, with the aim of preventing the onset of illness before a cure ever becomes necessary.

No one can stay well and healthy without the realization that we are made up not just of our bodies but of our minds and spirits too. When we find the right balance between these aspects of ourselves, all is well with us, whatever the circumstances. Bodily fitness and correct nutrition, vital as they are, will take us only so far. We also have to develop a positive mental attitude and an inner feeling of well-being if we are to really enjoy life. Total health has to be on all levels of consciousness. Fortunately, we can all achieve this for ourselves.

It is now accepted that the foods we eat play a large part in controlling whether or not we stay well and, perhaps also, happy. The most boring of sayings is 'You are what you eat,' and yet this has to be partly true. The problem is in knowing what we *should* eat. So much has been written on diet and vitamins that it might seem that there is nothing left to say: we should all be so fit and healthy.

We may know by heart the lists of the supposedly 'good' and 'bad' foods and the supplements that can cause unwelcome reactions for many. We are told that heart problems are more likely if one is overweight, yet many of the people one hears about or knows who have had a heart attack seem to be on the lean side. It must nevertheless be healthier – and certainly more comfortable – to carry less weight around.

I often wonder whether 'good' foods and 'bad' foods exist to the extent that we are led to believe. Surely, much depends on the effect that each food or combination of foods has on each of us as an individual. That is why awareness is so important: if a particular food you are eating doesn't feel right, then it probably isn't right – for *you*.

On the other hand – and this is where the difficulty comes in – many foods that are all right when eaten only occasionally are the very foods that are eaten by many in abundance. The so-called 'junk' foods – fast food, fried foods, confectionery and so on – do little harm if eaten once in a while, but to eat such foods as one's regular diet must be extremely harmful in the long run.

Whether dieting or not, it is essential to establish sensible, nutritious eating patterns, with adequate protein, fats and carbohydrates. Eating the *occasional* cream cake, dough-nut or whatever takes your fancy adds fun and enjoy-ment to life and must be fairly harmless. Such treats should remain occasional and not an everyday occur-rence, though.

At the same time, an over-restrictive way of eating will usually lead to cravings – and then binges. Strict diets – no chocolate allowed, for example – are fine for a while, but if you have a particular liking for chocolate you will probably end up eating it to excess at some later stage. Then all your resolutions go out of the window until the next 'I must lose weight' phase. Unless you have a consistent will of iron that enables you to maintain a strict eating regime, dieting will be a lifetime's pursuit.

For permanent success, whatever eating plan you choose

for yourself needs to be one that you enjoy and one that you can live with – one that includes the pleasure of meals with friends and family, without always having to prepare something different because everyone else is eating something that you are 'not allowed'. More or less any dieting plan will work for a while, but in the long run you will still have to learn how to eat all types of food without automatically putting on weight.

The answer is not to diet as such but to know when you have eaten enough and then stop eating. It is a simple method. Once you know that you can eat anything – that there are no 'guilty' foods – you can train yourself no longer to have those terrible cravings. You will be able to eat a reasonable amount of a previously forbidden food without feeling that you have done something wrong: without bingeing and then feeling 'What's the use?'

Let's see how we can take steps toward this.

1 Eat food that you enjoy. If this is solely 'junk' food – fried foods, biscuits, sugar and sweets – then you will have to take yourself in hand very seriously. Wide-ranging as one can be in one's choice of foods, a diet based solely on 'junk' foods cannot be good for you in the long run and will almost certainly be harmful – if not now, then in the future.

2 When you eat or drink, always taste and savour everything you put in your mouth. This may sound obvious, but many of us just look at our food – once it is in our mouths, we chew and swallow without paying much attention to its taste and texture.

This is almost always true of people with weight problems.

You will find that, by concentrating on what you are eating, you not only will enjoy your meals more but will also eat less.

Be aware that you are eating.

Be aware of what you are eating.

3 Between each mouthful, put your knife and fork, spoon, or whatever you are using, down on your plate. *Don't* pick them up again until you have savoured and swallowed the food in your mouth.

If you don't do this, you are likely to put more food in your mouth while you are still chewing the previous mouthful.

4 *When possible*, put your food on smaller plates. This really does give you the impression that you are eating more than is the case, and will leave you feeling just as satisfied.

5 When eating in restaurants, don't eat food you dislike just because you have paid for it. *Leave it* – otherwise you are treating yourself as a dustbin. Added to this, you will probably end up feeling ill.

6 Don't think of meals as having to consist of several courses. If one course is enough, then just eat that.

Learn to stop when you have eaten enough. That doesn't mean when you feel full: it means when your stomach has been satisfied, which is a very different feeling – one you will soon become aware of.

7 If you have a particular yearning for chocolate, then have some. But, here again, savour each piece and see how long you can make it last in your mouth before taking more – *if* you need it. Are you hungry after eating this chocolate? If not, then it has taken the place of a meal.

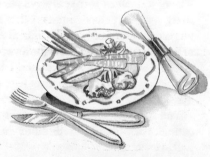

You don't have to eat by the clock: if you aren't hungry, don't eat. You can eat later, when you need food. *You won't starve.*

8 Don't deny yourself any particular foods that you enjoy. However, if they are of the cake or biscuit variety, don't buy any until this new way of eating becomes a habit. Once you have learned to control the way you eat, then you will be able to eat one cake, savour it, and possibly find it enough.

It's also important to plan meals that are nutritious, so that you don't need or want to fill up with desserts and biscuits.

9 Don't eat *anything* automatically. For example, don't automatically eat biscuits just because you have got into the habit of doing so when you have a cup of tea or coffee. Think before you put food in your mouth. Do you *really* feel hungry? If so, eat something with concentration on the content.

10 Don't eat to please others. This can be difficult if food has been prepared for you. If it's your family that's involved, make your new policy clear to them before any preparations go ahead.

11 Although you are not dieting here, eating less fat is always advisable. This does not mean *no fat* – some fat is essential for the body to function properly. But substitute vegetable-oil-based products for butter whenever you can, and cut down on other animal fats too, such as cream and full-fat milk as well as fatty meats.

12 High-fibre diets are now believed to be less healthful than first thought. Although it is important to have plenty of roughage, the fibre found in fruit and vegetables is sufficient and is certainly good for you.

13 Try cutting down on sugar and salt – these are both used unnecessarily a lot of the time. Each week, try to use a little less, then you won't notice the cut-back. After a

time, you may find that you don't need to use any at all.

14 Give up talking about diets and losing weight. This is like a red rag to a bull and always seems to lead to everyone insisting that you eat more than you want.

15 Finally, don't feel guilty about food: this often leads to secret bingeing. Just keep two things in mind: *eat only what you need* and *stop when you've eaten enough*.

The above is a way of eating for everyone – not just for those on a weight-loss diet.

If you *do* need to lose weight, however, you should decide for yourself how much *you* want to lose, instead of following the dictates of fashion. Even some of the 'ideal-weight' charts may not suit you.

Being very thin is not always attractive, and in some cases it can be harmful to one's health. In particular, as you get older, instead of looking slim there is a danger of looking just scrawny. This is never attractive. You need to feel comfortable about yourself. If this means weighing more than is specified by the magazines or whatever, then so be it. To be obese is certainly harmful, but to be slightly more ample than is fashionable can be attractive if it suits you and if you feel at ease like this.

I feel I should not end this section without mentioning the plight of factory-reared animals. In addition to the wretched conditions in which many of these are kept, there have been many articles and news reports on the dangers of produce from these sources – whether through contaminated feed, additives or antibiotics. This situation causes considerable concern to many of us.

It is important to be aware that there are farmers who rear their animals in a humane and natural environment, allowing them to graze and roam freely during their lifetime. The meat from these animals provides a healthier alternative to the drug-induced meat often found on display.

Many supermarkets now have organic meat as well as organic vegetables on sale, and at the end of the book, for those of you who are interested, I have given the address of the Soil Association, which maintains a list of suppliers of organic produce throughout the UK.

VITAMINS, MINERALS AND SUPPLEMENTS

Vitamins and minerals are essential for the healthy functioning of the body, but they cannot be made by the body itself and so they have to be provided in our diet. A balanced diet should provide all the vitamins and minerals that we need to keep ourselves in optimum health, and it is therefore essential to work out a nutritious eating plan with foods containing adequate amounts of these substances.

Although, in an ideal world, we should be able to get all our daily nutrients from the foods we eat, this is not always possible in practice. Not all vegetables are grown in soils containing the correct minerals, and the need for supermarkets to put food on sale in the best possible condition means that fruit cannot be left to sun-ripen. The resulting lack of naturally grown and ripened foods could leave us short of the vitamin and mineral intake we require, and it may then be necessary to take supplements to make up the deficiency. Although there are different schools of thought for and against the use of supplements, I feel that there are times when the body does need this additional assistance, at all ages.

Supplements can never take the place of nutritious foods, though. To eat 'junk' foods and then try to supplement them with vitamin capsules is not the route to healthy living or a happy existence.

Many articles in magazines and books advocate mega-doses of vitamin and mineral supplements, but I don't agree with this. Supplements can be as harmful as anything else if taken in excess.

For a complete nutritious diet, you need to eat a combination of foods which includes all of the vitamins and minerals described later. If you have any of the deficiency symptoms listed, try increasing your intake of the appropriate food(s) before resorting to a supplement of any kind.

When adding supplements to your diet, it is better to take a multivitamin and multimineral supplement, so as not to cause an imbalance in your system. If you feel that you are particularly deficient in any one substance, it is advisable to consult a doctor or nutritionist knowledgeable in vitamin and mineral supplementation.

The quality of supplements varies, and it is important to buy from a reliable source.

The water-soluble vitamins (see below) pass through the system fairly rapidly, so it is better to take these – especially vitamins B and C – at intervals throughout the day. An alternative is to take a time-release supplement. This releases the vitamins gradually, ensuring absorption in the body over a period of up to twelve hours.

It is better to take supplements with a main meal – either as part of or after the meal.

There are two broad classes of vitamins: fat-soluble and water-soluble.

The fat-soluble vitamins are vitamins A, D, E, F and K. These vitamins are stored in the body, and they can therefore build up to toxic levels if they are taken in large doses over a long period.

The water-soluble vitamins are vitamins B, C and P (bioflavonoids). These vitamins are not stored in the body, so a daily intake is essential. Any excess intake of water-soluble vitamins is excreted.

When taking vitamin supplements, it is important to note the quantities concerned.

Quantities of fat-soluble vitamins – that is, vitamins A, D, E, F and K – are measured in international units (IU).

Quantities of water-soluble vitamins are usually measured in milligrams (mg).

Quantities of some vitamins and minerals are measured in smaller units – micrograms (mcg).

VITAMINS

VITAMIN A

Properties
- Essential for the health of the skin – lack of this vitamin can lead to dry, scaly skin and blemishes.
- Builds resistance to infections of the mucous membrane – catarrh and bronchial complaints.
- Promotes healthy hair, teeth and gums.
- Helps in the treatment of many eye disorders – a deficiency in vitamin A can result in impaired vision at night.

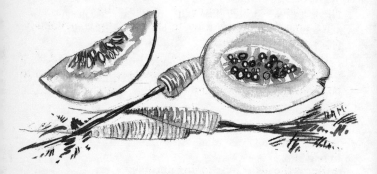

Food Sources Vitamin A is found in different forms in plants and animals. The plant form, which is known as beta-carotene, is stored in the body and is converted to vitamin A as it is needed. Beta-carotene is not toxic and can be taken in larger doses without ill effects. This form, rather than vitamin A derived from fish-liver oil, say, is recommended for women during pregnancy.

- Plant sources – carrots, green and yellow vegetables, yellow fruits, dried apricots, papayas, cantaloup melons
- Animal sources – fish-liver oils, liver

Recommended Daily Allowance   5,000 to 10,000 IU
With an adequate intake of the above foods, you should not need a vitamin-A supplement. If a supplement is needed, though, for proper absorption of vitamin A it should be taken with B-complex vitamins, vitamin E, calcium and zinc.

B-COMPLEX VITAMINS

These vitamins are water-soluble, so a daily intake is needed.

All B vitamins are essential for the health of the nervous system.

They also ensure proper utilization of carbohydrates, fats and proteins essential for healthy skin and hair.

Vitamin B-deficiency leads to chronic fatigue, irritability, depression and indigestion.

Details of individual B vitamins are given below, but, if supplements are required, the B-complex vitamins need to be taken as a whole and not as single B vitamins.

VITAMIN B1 (THIAMINE)

Properties
- Keeps the heart functioning normally.
- Improves digestion and assimilation of foods – especially starches, sugars and alcohol.
- Essential for proper functioning of the nervous system.

Food Sources   Fresh vegetables, wheatgerm, wholewheat, potatoes, beans, peanuts, dried yeast, pork

Recommended Daily Allowance   1 to 1.2 mg
Heavy drinkers or smokers need to increase their intake of
this vitamin.

VITAMIN B2 (RIBOFLAVIN)

Properties
- Promotes healthy skin, hair, nails and eyes – deficiency
  in this vitamin leads to cracks and sores around the
  mouth and poor vision.
- Increases overall vitality and stamina.

Food Sources   Leafy green vegetables, yeast, wheatgerm,
peanuts, soya beans, cheese, milk, eggs, liver, kidney,
fish

Recommended Daily Allowance   1.6 mg

VITAMIN B3
(NIACIN, NIACINAMIDE, NICOTINAMIDE)

Properties
- Improves circulation and reduces high blood pressure.
- Helps the proper functioning of the central nervous
  system.
- Maintains the health of the skin, tongue and digestive-
  system tissue.
- Helps to prevent or eases the effects of migraine head-
  aches.
- Is used in the treatment of pellagra.
- Is beneficial in the treatment of schizophrenia.

In some cases, niacin can cause temporary flushing or
itching of the skin. This side-effect is not serious and wears
off quickly. Niacinamide (nicotinamide) – the synthetic
form of vitamin B3 – does not cause this effect.

Food Sources   Whole grains, wheatgerm, soya beans, nuts, dates, figs, avocados, fish, poultry, liver, kidney

Recommended Daily Allowance   12 to 18 mg (50 to 100 mg more usual)

VITAMIN B5
(PANTOTHENIC ACID, CALCIUM PANTOTHENATE)

Properties
- Stimulates the adrenal glands – important for healthy nerves and skin.
- Helps prevent constipation and other digestive disorders.
- Helpful in the relief of allergies, if combined with vitamin C.
- Helps relieve stress.
- Reduces toxic effects when on antibiotics.

Food Sources   Green vegetables, wheatgerm, whole grains, dried beans, nuts, poultry, liver, kidney, heart

Recommended Daily Allowance   10 mg (10 to 100 mg more usual)

VITAMIN B6 (PYRIDOXINE)

Properties
- Helpful during premenstrual tension and incidences of water retention.
- Deficiency symptoms include insomnia, muscle spasms, cramp and numbness.
- Promotes normal functioning of the nervous system.

Food Sources   Brown rice, whole grains, wheatgerm, milk, eggs, bananas, seeds, fish, beef, liver, kidney

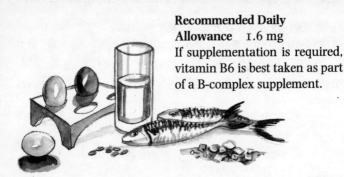

Recommended Daily Allowance 1.6 mg
If supplementation is required, vitamin B6 is best taken as part of a B-complex supplement.

VITAMIN B12 (CYANOCOBALAMIN)

Quantities of this vitamin are measured in micrograms (mcg).

Properties
- Helps overcome disorders of the nervous system.
- Reduces fatigue, irritability, insomnia, inability to concentrate and lack of balance.

Food Sources Liver, kidney, beef, eggs, milk, cheese, fish, wheatgerm

Recommended Daily Allowance 3 mcg
Vegetarians may have a particular need to supplement vitamin B12. Vitamin B6 is needed for proper absorption of this vitamin.

BIOTIN (VITAMIN H – PART OF THE B COMPLEX)

Quantities of this vitamin are measured in micrograms (mcg).

Properties
- Helps utilization of protein, folic acid and vitamin B12.
- Maintains healthy skin and hair.

- A strong cell-growth stimulant.
- Deficiency in biotin can cause muscle cramps and anaemia.

Food Sources Fruits, nuts, egg yolk, milk, brown rice, liver, kidney

Recommended Daily Allowance 50 to 300 mcg

CHOLINE (PART OF THE B COMPLEX)

Properties
- Prevents fats accumulating in the liver.
- Vital for proper nerve–muscle function.
- Helps the memory – used in the treatment of Alzheimer's disease.
- Helps regulate and improve liver and gall-bladder functioning.

Food Sources Dried yeast, egg yolk, liver, kidney, lecithin

Recommended Daily Allowance Not established (usually 50 mg)

FOLIC ACID (PART OF THE B COMPLEX)

Quantities of this vitamin are measured in micrograms (mcg).

Properties
- Essential for formation of red blood cells.
- Used to treat some forms of anaemia.

Food Sources Green vegetables, carrots, yellow fruits, avocados, wholewheat, beans, egg yolk, liver, brewer's yeast

Recommended Daily Allowance 400 mcg

INOSITOL (PART OF THE B COMPLEX)

Properties
- Helps in removing fats from the liver to the cells.
- Vital for the health of hair and hair growth.
- Protects the liver, kidneys and heart.
- Helps prevent eczema.
- Helpful in brain-cell nutrition.

Food Sources   Whole grains, brown rice, dried beans, raisins, grapefruit, peanuts, beef heart, lecithin

Recommended Daily Allowance   Not established (usually 250 to 500 mg)
Inositol should be combined with choline to form lecithin. Lecithin itself is available in powder and granule form to add to liquids.

PBA (PARA-AMINOBENZOIC ACID – PART OF THE B COMPLEX)

Properties
- Aids the formation of red blood cells.
- Stimulates intestinal bacteria to produce folic acid.
- Keeps skin healthy.
- Important to hair pigmentation – when used with folic acid and vitamin B5, it helps to restore hair to its natural colour.
- Used as an ointment to protect skin from sunburn.

Food Sources   Brown rice, yeast, wheatgerm, whole grains, liver, kidney

Recommended Daily Allowance   Not established (usually 30 to 100 mg)

VITAMIN C (ASCORBIC ACID)

Properties
- Helps in production of collagen – the protein necessary for the formation of connective tissue in skin, ligaments and bones.
- Speeds the healing of wounds.
- Helps the formation of red blood cells.
- Fights bacterial infection.

Food Sources
Potatoes, citrus fruits, rosehips, berries, tomatoes, green vegetables (especially broccoli), green peppers

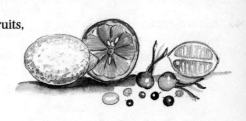

Recommended Daily Allowance   45 mg (500 to 1,000 mg more usual)
Vitamin C is a water-soluble nutrient, which means that it quickly flows through the digestive tract and out in the urine. So, if supplementation is required, vitamin C should be taken throughout the day, rather than in large single doses.

Extra vitamin C is advisable for smokers, aspirin-takers and women on the pill.

Yoghurt can decrease the absorption of this vitamin.

VITAMIN D

Properties
- Helps maintain a stable nervous system.
- Helps the absorption and distribution of calcium – essential for healthy bone and tooth formation.

Food Sources Milk and dairy products, egg yolk, fish-liver oils, mackerel, herring, salmon, sardines

Recommended Daily Allowance 400 IU
Vitamin D is a fat-soluble vitamin, so it is stored in the body, unlike the water-soluble vitamins B and C.

Vitamin D can be made in the skin with the presence of sunlight, so the amount of any supplementation needed will depend on your exposure to sunlight – in the winter, you would obviously need more.

VITAMIN E (TOCOPHEROLS)

Vitamin E consists of a group of substances called tocopherols. The most active of these is alpha tocopherol, and this is preferable to the mixed tocopherols.

Properties
- Helps protect vitamin A and B-complex vitamins from destruction in the body.
- Increases endurance and stamina.
- Increases the blood flow to the heart and throughout the body.
- Prevents blood-clot formation.
- Slows down the ageing process in cells.

Food Sources Wheatgerm, whole grains, wholewheat, green vegetables, soya beans, cold-pressed vegetable oils, eggs, seeds

Recommended Daily Allowance 15 to 30 IU

VITAMIN F (UNSATURATED FATTY ACIDS – LINOLEIC, LINOLENIC AND ARACHIDONIC ACIDS)

Properties
- Essential for normal glandular activity.

- Prevents the nails becoming brittle.
- Promotes healthy skin and hair – deficiency in this vitamin can cause dandruff, eczema, acne, dry skin and allergies.
- Helps to reduce cholesterol deposits.

Food Sources Cod-liver oil, lecithin, sunflower and linseed oils, soya beans, seeds, avocados, almonds, peanuts, walnuts

Recommended Daily Allowance Not established (food sources should be adequate)
For better absorption, vitamin E should be taken with this vitamin.

VITAMIN K

Properties
- Essential for blood clotting.
- Helps reduce heavy periods.
- Helps proper liver functioning.

Food Sources Yoghurt (acidophilus culture), green vegetables, kelp, egg yolk, fish-liver oils

Recommended Daily Allowance Not established (food sources should be adequate)

VITAMIN P (BIOFLAVONOIDS, CITRUS BIOFLAVONOIDS, RUTIN, HESPERIDIN)

Properties
- Essential for the proper absorption and functioning of vitamin C.
- Helps vitamin C in the production and maintenance of collagen.
- Increases capillary strength – helping to prevent haemorrhages, bleeding gums, varicose veins and severe bruising.

Food Sources Concentrated in the pulpy white part o
citrus fruits, apricots, blackberries, cherries

Recommended Daily Allowance Not established (usuall
100 mg of vitamin P to every 500 mg of vitamin C)

MINERALS

CALCIUM

Properties

- Essential, with
  phosphorus, for the
  health of teeth and
  bones.
- Essential, with
  magnesium, for
  heart and muscle
  functioning.
- Helps prevent
  backache and
  period pains.
- Taken at night,
  helps relaxation.

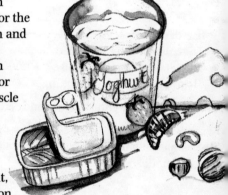

Food Sources Milk, yoghurt, cheese, whole grains, gree
vegetables, kelp, sardines, salmon, nuts, seeds, dried beans

Recommended Daily Allowance 800 to 1,200 mg

COPPER

Properties

- Helps the formation of red blood cells.

- With vitamin C, helps the formation of elastin, the chief component of elastic muscle fibre in the body.

Food Sources Whole grains, wholewheat, dried beans, peas, kelp, seafood, liver

Recommended Daily Allowance Supplies of copper in food and water are considered adequate and supplementation is not usually advisable.

IODINE

Quantities of this mineral are measured in micrograms (mcg).

Properties
- Essential for the development and functioning of the thyroid gland.
- Promotes healthy hair, skin, nails and teeth.
- Stimulates the metabolism, helping the body to burn off excess fat.

Food Sources Kelp, onions, seafood, seaweed

Recommended Daily Allowance 100 mcg
Supplementation is not usually necessary.

IRON

Properties
- Increases resistance to stress and disease, especially anaemia.
- Prevents fatigue.
- Helps metabolize A, B-complex and C vitamins.

Food Sources Dried apricots and peaches, raisins, leafy green vegetables, asparagus, nuts, oatmeal, red meat, liver, kidney, heart

Recommended Daily Allowance 18 mg

The following are required for utilization of iron: vitamin C, copper, manganese, folic acid, calcium, phosphorus and cobalt.

Avoid ferrous-sulphate iron supplements. Ferrous gluconate or citrate iron are preferable, as they do not neutralize vitamin E.

Like other supplements, iron should be taken with food, but it is best not to take iron supplements at a meal when you are eating cereals, as fibre inhibits its absorption. For better absorption, take iron with milk, vitamin C or citrus fruits.

MAGNESIUM

Properties

- Promotes absorption and metabolism of calcium, phosphorus, sodium, potassium, and vitamins B6, C and D.
- Helps bone growth.
- Necessary for the proper functioning of the nerves and muscles, especially of the heart.
- Helps the body to utilize fats, proteins and carbohydrates.
- Helps prevent kidney stones and gall stones.

Food Sources Green vegetables, soya beans, almonds, corn, celery, brown rice, seeds, apples, grapefruit, lemons, figs

Recommended Daily Allowance 300 mg

MANGANESE

Properties

- Necessary for proper glandular functioning, especially sex-hormone production.

- Nourishes nerves and the brain – improves memory.
- Reduces nervous irritability.

Food Sources Leafy green vegetables, dried beans, peas, beets, egg yolk, whole grains

Recommended Daily Allowance Not established (usually 3 to 7 mg)
Manganese is most effective when taken with vitamins B1, C and E.

PHOSPHORUS

Properties
- Helps in the maintenance and repair of cells.
- Helps utilize carbohydrates, fats and proteins.
- Helps promote healthy teeth and gums.
- Helps promote proper kidney functioning.

Food Sources Meat, fish, poultry, eggs, whole grains, nuts, seeds

Recommended Daily Allowance 800 to 1,200 mg
Phosphorus is absorbed best when taken with calcium, manganese, and vitamins A and D.

POTASSIUM

Properties
- Stimulates the kidneys to eliminate toxic body wastes.
- Helps prevent stress and premenstrual tension.
- Promotes healthy skin.

Food Sources Citrus fruits, leafy green vegetables, figs, bananas, potatoes, seeds

Recommended Daily Allowance Not established (usually 900 mg)

If you drink a lot of coffee or alcohol, you may need to increase your intake of food rich in this mineral.

When taking diuretics, the loss of potassium can be considerable, and some diuretics now contain this mineral to compensate.

SELENIUM

Quantities of this mineral are measured in micrograms.

Properties
- Works together with vitamin E in promoting good body growth and fertility.
- Helps preserve the elasticity of tissue.
- Helpful in the treatment of dandruff.
- Can lessen the effect of menopausal symptoms.

Food Sources Wheatgerm, broccoli, tomatoes, onions, garlic, tuna fish

Recommended Daily Allowance Not established (usually 50 to 100 mcg)

ZINC

Properties
- Speeds the healing of wounds and burns.
- Eliminates white spots on the fingernails.
- Necessary for the growth and development of the reproductive organs.
- Can be helpful in cases of irregular periods.
- Assists absorption of vitamins, especially B-complex vitamins.

Food Sources High-protein foods: beef, lamb, pork, seafood, brewer's yeast, eggs, seeds

Recommended Daily Allowance   15 mg
Zinc is most effective when taken with vitamin A, calcium
and phosphorus.

LOOKING AFTER YOUR HANDS AND NAILS

Looking after your hands and nails need not take up very much of your time, but it is essential to keep up a fairly regular routine if you want permanent results.

- Keep a pot of hand cream in the bathroom and kitchen. It takes only seconds to massage a little cream into your hands and nails when you need to.
- Wear cotton household gloves for any rough work.
- Wear gardening gloves for any gardening jobs.
- Wear rubber gloves when using strong detergents.

Keep your gloves handy for wherever you are likely to use them, and get into the habit of putting them on – it is worth while.

- Massage your hands with slightly damp salt. This will help to remove dead skin and to keep your hands smooth. The backs of your hands are particularly important here.
- Before you go to bed at night, massage your nails with good cuticle and nail cream. The base of the nail is very important here. As the nail grows, it will then be more flexible, less brittle, less inclined to break or flake.
- Be careful how you file your nails. Always file from the side of the nail to the centre. This will prevent your nail from splitting. Never file backwards and forwards in a sawing movement – it may be easier, but your nails will split or flake.

  When you finish, seal the edges of your nails by lightly going over the tips with the emery board, using with a downward movement towards the palm.

- Be careful to be very gentle with the base of the nail, round the cuticle. It is very easy to damage the nail here.
- If your nails are in poor condition and you are not exposing them to strong detergents and so on, then your diet may be at fault. Eat foods rich in the B vitamins (see page 159) to help your nails grow strong and healthy.
- Treat yourself to a professional manicure. This is really worthwhile if you need to improve the appearance of your nails quickly. Don't worry about presenting a manicurist with nails that look *really* awful. That's when you most need help, and a good manicurist will love the challenge. Just one visit will show you how to care for your nails more quickly than reading about it.

You will need to keep up your own good work regularly, though, or you will be back to square one quicker than you think.

Many women are very concerned about brown spots on the backs of their hands. These are sometimes referred to as 'liver' spots, although they have nothing to do with the liver – I can only think they are called this because of their colour.

The main cause of these spots is apparently too much exposure to the sun. They can also appear on the face and other parts of the body, though they are usually less noticeable there and of course can more easily be masked by cosmetics. A precaution could be always to wear a sunscreen product on the hands during the summer. Even wear cotton gloves if you are very prone to this problem, especially when driving – the sun through the windscreen can be particularly powerful.

There are creams on the market which are supposed to gradually fade out these spots. I have not had cause to try out these products, but I have been told that they take a long time to have any effect, and even then they may not be that successful. These creams contain a bleaching agent which is fairly strong and in some cases can cause allergic reactions. It cannot be a good idea to use any products containing strong chemicals, so if only for caution on health grounds I would advise against this method.

If you are really concerned about them, these spots can be removed professionally, through skin-peeling and other similar methods. I have known only two clients who have had such treatment. One was delighted, the other said 'never again'. If you *are* investigating the various treatments, though, do ask if there are any side-effects, pigmentation problems, or possible scarring. Practitioners should tell you this – if they don't, you must ask.

B-complex vitamins in supplements, together with a nutritious diet, are thought to prevent and, in milder cases, to cure this problem.

Exercising the arms, hands and fingers will help to prevent stiff joints and will give your hands a better appearance. If your joints are already stiff, they will gradually become more flexible, but you will need to work fairly gently – just a few movements a day without strain is best.

Stiff and/or swollen joints can be caused through one's diet. It is worthwhile to check your food intake when any stiffness seems especially pronounced. In my case, the joints of my right hand become swollen when I eat oranges. A doctor friend says, 'Most unlikely.' I say, 'It does seem unlikely, but nevertheless it is true.'

On the following pages you will find some hand exercises that you can do at any time – while travelling, waiting for someone, watching television or in bed. Remember never to use force with these exercises – or any others for that matter. With exercise, the flexibility and general improvement and appearance of your hands will become apparent in a very short time, so do work out daily – if only briefly.

TO INCREASE CIRCULATION

1 Place the palms of your hands
together, fingers facing upwards.

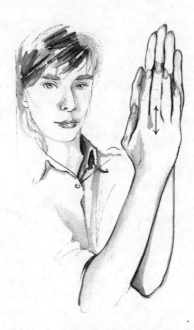

2 Now rub the palms of your hands,
including your wrists, together briskly
for at least 10 seconds.

3 Follow by shaking out your hands,
keeping your wrists limp.

Do this again later, while you are doing
your hand exercises.

FOR SUPPLENESS OF THE FINGERS AND HANDS

1 Press your hands together, fingers facing upwards, your elbows out at the sides.

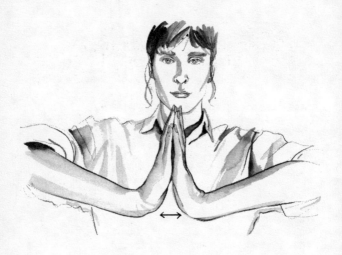

2 Keeping your fingers pointing straight upwards, bend your hands back at the lower knuckles so that your palms move away from each other.

3 Hold for a count of five.

Relax and shake out your hands.

If flexible enough, do this three times.

FOR FLEXIBILITY OF THE FINGERS

In turn, bend each finger at the two
different joints.

1 Curl each finger over and press at the
top joint (as in the illustration), then
straighten the finger.

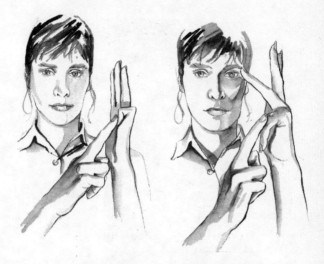

2 Then bend in turn each straight finger
towards the palm. Press gently on the
finger near the knuckle (as in the
illustration).

This exercise helps the energy in the
fingers and joints to flow more freely.

> *If your joints are stiff, work very gently
> with all these exercises. Do not use force.*

TO LOOSEN STIFF FINGERS

1 Hold one hand in front of you at chest level, palm down.

2 With the thumb of your other hand, raise each finger in turn backwards.

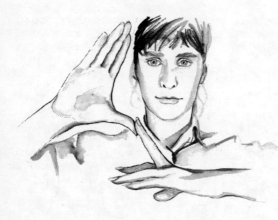

The raised finger should be at right angles to your hand.

3 Repeat with the other hand.

Shake out your arms, wrists and hands vigorously.

> *Your fingers may be too stiff to be bent back so far. If so, don't worry – and don't use force. Your fingers will gradually become more flexible.*

FOR GENERAL CIRCULATION AND FLEXIBILITY OF THE JOINTS

Stand with your feet slightly apart, your arms at your sides. (If you prefer, you can do this exercise sitting down.)

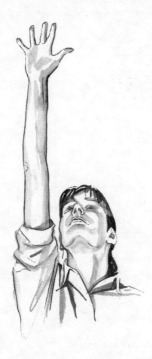

1 Stretch your right arm over your head as far as possible.

2 Now spread your fingers wide apart and look up at your hand. Really stretch up.

3 Now relax your right arm at your side.

4 Repeat with your left arm.

5 Now stretch up with both arms, stretching the fingers wide apart.

6 Relax both arms at your sides.

Do this three times.

Really stretch up each time.

When you have finished this exercise, bend forward and relax. Then shake your arms and shoulders.

FOR SUPPLENESS OF THE FINGERS AND HANDS

1 Spread out the fingers of both hands.

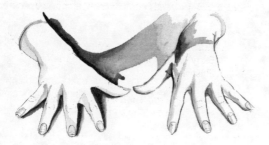

2 Then make a fist.

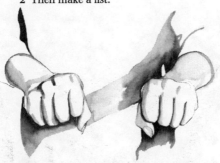

3 Spread out the fingers, then make a fist again.

Repeat these movements twenty times.

Shake out your hands and relax them.

> *Be careful your nails don't dig into your palms here.*

HAND MASSAGE

Massaging the hands for a minute or two each day is very stimulating for the whole body as well as keeping your hands in better condition. The circulation in your hands and fingers will improve enormously.

1 Hold one hand with the other, in a fairly relaxed way, as shown in the illustration.

2 Now, with the thumb, massage your hand all over. Start at the fingertips and work down.

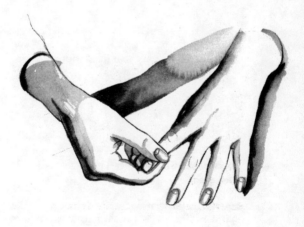

Keep your neck, shoulders and arms relaxed throughout.

HAND MASSAGE

3 Massage your palm and your thumb joint.

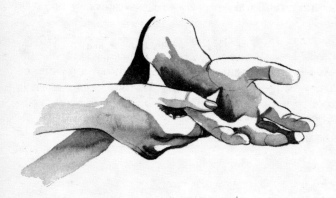

4 Massage the sides of your hand with a gentle pinching movement.

5 Now turn your hand over and repeat in the same way.

6 Massage all round the wrist.

Do the same with the other hand.

You can do this massage at any time – in bed, while travelling or when waiting for someone. Make this a daily habit.

> *Don't frown or squint.*
> *This applies all the time – even here.*

ALTERNATIVE WAYS TO <u>*HEALTH*</u>

I would like to introduce you to a few alternative therapies for better health. Some of you will already have heard of these or may even have experience of them. However, if you haven't come across these techniques before, or if you would like a brief reminder about them, this section is for you. I must point out, though, that I am not a consultant in any of these methods, but I consider them of such potential value that it is worth bringing them to your attention.

First you will find a brief description of the McTimoney Chiropractic Method. This is a gentle, effective and safe means of realigning the bones of the body when they have become displaced, whether after injury or just through the wear and tear of everyday living.

Secondly, the Alexander Technique. Again, this method has to do with the correct relationship of the different parts of the body in everyday situations. The joy of this method is that it does not dictate rigid rules about posture but teaches the *individual* to use his or her body in the most natural way.

Finally, there is an outline of the technique of reflexology, or zone therapy, which originated in China and Egypt about 2,500 years BC, making it possibly one of the oldest therapies known.

These three different methods all share the belief that it is essential to treat the body as a whole, not just the obvious areas in pain, thus giving the opportunity for total healing.

Many of us wait until we suffer considerable pain before we consult a practitioner. Of course, pain does sometimes go away through the body having made the necessary adjustments itself, but it is unwise to wait too long in the hope that this will happen.

Obviously, prevention of damage should be our main concern, and the way we use our bodies in everyday living is of the utmost importance. When the work of supporting and moving the body is being wrongly distributed, we are putting ourselves under tremendous strain and could even be impairing bodily functions such as the circulation of the blood and breathing patterns. Such malfunctions can lead to chronic fatigue and a general feeling of not being as well as one could be.

THE McTIMONEY CHIROPRACTIC METHOD

I have chosen to describe the McTimoney method rather than other chiropractic techniques of equal effectiveness because it is an extremely gentle approach.

The technique was developed by John McTimoney, who was trained by Dr Mary Walker, DC, a graduate of the first chiropractic college to be established – Palmer College, in Iowa, USA. John McTimoney later refined and extended his training into a total chiropractic method which integrated the whole body structurally.

His approach was based on the belief that the main cause of disease and pain is the misalignment of the bones. The backbone, or spine, tends to take the brunt of our everyday stresses and strains. As a result, some bones may move slightly out of their correct position.

Apart from being our framework, our bones also act as packaging to protect delicate organs, blood vessels, nerves, etc. In particular, a delicate thread of fibres which makes up the spinal cord or column runs through the segments of bone (called vertebrae) which make up the spine. From the spinal cord, nerves branch off to act as communication lines to relay messages to and from the brain.

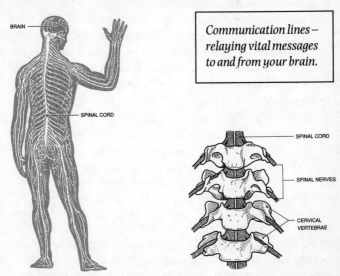

Communication lines – relaying vital messages to and from your brain.

When one or more of the vertebrae becomes misaligned, the resulting pressure on the spinal cord can cause problems. Not only will there be pain in the back itself, other parts of the body will also not be working as well as they should be, because their nerves from the spinal cord may have been affected too. In many cases, inflammation and swelling around the nerves may cause considerable restriction of movement and intense discomfort.

A practitioner of the McTimoney Chiropractic Method will adjust the vertebrae back into the right place, releasing the pressure that causes inflammation and allowing normal functioning to resume.

Having corrected the spine, the same attention is given to other joints in the body, including your ankles, elbows and knees, to make sure that every nerve is free to work properly.

THE ALEXANDER TECHNIQUE

I have often noticed that people in their later years who are very upright in stature, rather than stooped, appear to remain more active, supple and alert in every way, so it seems worthwhile to study ways in which to achieve this. One way is the Alexander Technique.

An interesting observation which stemmed from my study of the Alexander Technique is that many of us seem to be trying to contract our bodies – and indeed our whole being – for example by seeming to contract our head towards our trunk. By doing the opposite – by feeling an expansion of our being – our outlook on life can be transformed. It seems so simple and obvious, but our posture really is of great importance, not least in conveying our state of mind to others.

The Alexander Technique was devised in the early part of this century by Frederic Matthias Alexander. He was an actor, in Australia, who was having difficulties with his speech. When doctors and specialists could find no organic reasons for these difficulties, he decided that the cause must be what he came to describe as 'misuse of the self', through almost complete ignorance of the correct way in which to use the body.

A central principle of Alexander's teaching is the importance of the relationship between the head, the neck and the back. For example, habits such as holding the head contracted backwards and downwards may over the years result in a compression of the spine which eventually interferes with the muscular and nervous system.

If something is wrong with us, the usual response is to think we must do something about the symptoms. Alexander, however, believed that if something is wrong with us then we should find out what is causing the problem and stop doing it. I find this a very interesting way of thinking.

When you sit or stand in a slumped position, the pressure on your internal organs prevents them from functioning properly. In particular, the pressure on the spine when it is unevenly loaded by poor posture can lead to pressure on the nerves and malfunctioning of other parts of the body, as we saw when we looked at the McTimoney Chiropractic Method. But simply sitting or standing up straight is not the answer. What is needed is a method of moving which prevents tension anywhere in the body but brings about ease throughout. It is this method that the Alexander Technique teaches you.

The basic movement consists in always letting your head ease up first when moving from any position and letting the body follow. Many of us do the opposite – first contracting into ourselves in order to stand up, for example.

As an example, try turning your head from side to side now. I am sure that many of you will have contracted your head downwards into the trunk of your body as you did this. Now try turning your head to the left or the right while at the same time lifting your head up and away from your body so that your neck extends and your body follows the upward movement of the head. Even if not turning your body, it should automatically tend to ease upwards.

As a final example, look up at the ceiling. You will probably find that you have contracted your head towards your shoulders to do this. Try again, this time easing your head up and then tilting it towards the ceiling.

We often move our heads by leading with the chin, which automatically tends to draw the head downwards towards the body. It is better to think of your head as one unit and to move it as one, with ease.

I have obviously given only a very brief idea of this method, and you would need to know very much more about this subtle technique before starting to move in this new way. There are many books on the subject; however, if you find it of interest, I think it is important to contact a trained Alexander teacher, who can teach you how to make the technique work best for *you*. Age is no barrier to taking up the Alexander Technique – even after many years of misusing your body, you can still bring about very beneficial changes – but it is a technique to be used throughout one's life, so it seems advisable to get it right.

REFLEXOLOGY

A totally different type of therapy is reflexology – or zone therapy.

This method is based on the concept of a system of channels which carry energy through the body, with main channels or zones to every part of us – our nerves, organs, glands and so on.

These zones were first brought to the attention of the Western medical world by an American specialist, Dr William Fitzgerald, in the 1930s. Dr Fitzgerald described the existence of ten longitudinal zones in the body and developed a form of treatment based on these, which he called zone therapy.

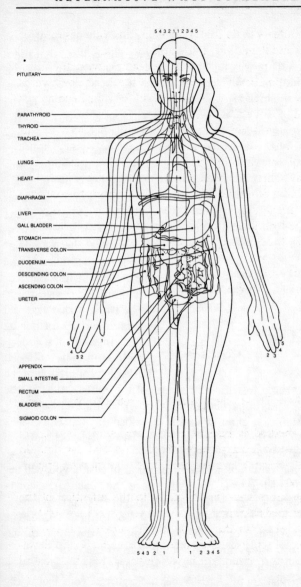

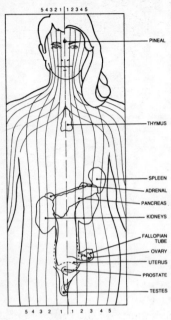

If you look at the illustrations, you will see that these zones run straight through the body. Each zone runs from a particular toe to the head and then down to the corresponding finger. For example, zone 1 is everything in line with the big toe, running up through the body to the head and then down the arm in line with the thumb. During treatment, pressure is applied at a point in a zone to influence the energy flow in that particular channel.

The work of Dr Fitzgerald was later carried further by Eunice Ingham, an American physiotherapist. She felt that benefit could be obtained by working just the extremities of the zones – that is, the hands and, in particular, the feet – with the same effect. It was Eunice Ingham who first described the pattern of reflex points in the feet on which is based the technique of reflexology as it is known today.

If you now look at the illustration opposite, you will see a map of the feet. You will notice that each area corresponds to a part of the body. The right foot corresponds to the right side of the body; the left foot to the left side. The narrowest part of the foot, about halfway down, is equivalent to the waistline. So, the area from the centre of your foot to the toes represents the top part of your body – from your waistline upwards. From the centre of your foot to the

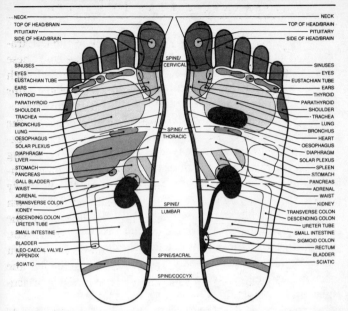

heel represents the lower part of your body – from your waistline down.

The reflex areas are not only found on the soles, but also on the sides and the tops of the feet.

To give a brief summary:

- The big-toe areas correspond to the head and brain.
- The front of the big toe corresponds to the face.
- The little toes correspond to the sinuses and teeth.
- The eye reflexes are found just beneath the second and third toes.
- The spine reflex is found down the inner sides of both feet, since the spine is situated centrally in the body.
- The lung areas are found over the balls of the feet.
- Digestive areas are found below waist level on both feet.
- Joints – including shoulders, elbows, knees and hips – are found on the outer sides of both feet.
- The lymphatic system is found on the tops of both feet.

Reflexology is thought to stimulate the individual's own healing capabilities, encouraging the body to put itself right more quickly. With many disorders, the healing forces at work result in recovery occurring without medication.

Although there are many self-treatment books on reflexology, it is considered advisable to have treatment with a qualified practitioner – at least to start with.

Although the method may seem quite simple – just applying pressure on the various reflex points – it is possible for strong reactions to occur. The massage should be applied to the reflex points very carefully; the pressure used is not severe. If reflex areas are overworked, by applying too much pressure, or by working on the reflex points, it is possible to cause unpleasant reactions in the body.

Having treatment at weekly intervals will prevent overworking, as well as giving the body a chance to put itself right in the meantime. Overworking will not generally cause irreversible damage, in fact, but it is unnecessary to cause such a reaction in the first place.

In addition to the reflex areas found in the feet, similar points are found in the hands. The hands are obviously a more easily accessible area for self-treatment and may be used for the treatment and relief of individual symptoms. The arrangement of the reflex points is similar, with the presence of the same ten longitudinal zones. Remember, though, that the reflexes in the hands can also be overworked, so care should be taken here too.

Reflexology is a treatment which can be used on all age groups and for the majority of conditions. Many people will completely recover from their disorder; others will see a great improvement. Some – especially those with serious disorders – may not notice a great improvement in specific symptoms but may nevertheless feel better in themselves and thus be more able to cope.

In all instances, treatment should lead to improved

functioning of all the body's eliminating systems, enabling toxins to be cleared from the system rather than just collecting in the body and causing further problems.

Also, the treatment can be very effective in relieving pain. The feeling of well-being and relaxation experienced by nearly everyone who has tried this treatment is in itself a great encouragement in promoting healing and better health.

Eva Fraser
Facial Workout Studio
Enquiries Tel: 0181 789-3612

The Soil Association (Organic Produce)
86 Colston Street
Bristol BS1 5BB Tel: 0117 9290661

Cosmetics à la Carte Tel: 0171 622-2318

Your True Colours Ltd Tel: 0171 435-0726

Colour Me Beautiful Tel: 0171 627-5211

The Institute of Pure Chiropractic
14 Park End Street
Oxford OX1 1HH Tel: 01865 246687

Society of Teachers of the Alexander
   Technique
20 London House
266 Fulham Road
London SW10 9EL Tel: 0171 351-0828

The British Reflexology Association
Monks Orchard
Whitbourne
Worcester WR6 5RB Tel: 01886 21207

Nicola Hall
Bayley School of Reflexology
Monks Orchard
Whitbourne
Worcester WR6 5RB Tel: 01886 21207

Discover more about our forthcoming books through Penguin's FREE newspaper...

Penguin

Quarterly

It's packed with:

- exciting features
- author interviews
- previews & reviews
- books from your favourite films & TV series
- exclusive competitions & much, much more...

READ MORE IN PENGUIN

In every corner of the world, on every subject under the sun, Penguin represents quality and variety – the very best in publishing today.

For complete information about books available from Penguin – including Puffins, Penguin Classics and Arkana – and how to order them, write to us at the appropriate address below. Please note that for copyright reasons the selection of books varies from country to country.

In the United Kingdom: Please write to *Dept. JC, Penguin Books Ltd, FREEPOST, West Drayton, Middlesex UB7 OBR.*

If you have any difficulty in obtaining a title, please send your order with the correct money, plus ten per cent for postage and packaging, to *PO Box No. 11, West Drayton, Middlesex UB7 OBR*

In the United States: Please write to *Consumer Sales, Penguin USA, P.O. Box 999, Dept. 17109, Bergenfield, New Jersey 07621-0120.* VISA and MasterCard holders call 1-800-253-6476 to order all Penguin titles

In Canada: Please write to *Penguin Books Canada Ltd, 10 Alcorn Avenue, Suite 300, Toronto, Ontario M4V 3B2*

In Australia: Please write to *Penguin Books Australia Ltd, P.O. Box 257, Ringwood, Victoria 3134*

In New Zealand: Please write to *Penguin Books (NZ) Ltd, Private Bag 102902, North Shore Mail Centre, Auckland 10*

In India: Please write to *Penguin Books India Pvt Ltd, 706 Eros Apartments, 56 Nehru Place, New Delhi 110 019*

In the Netherlands: Please write to *Penguin Books Netherlands bv, Postbus 3507, NL-1001 AH Amsterdam*

In Germany: Please write to *Penguin Books Deutschland GmbH, Metzlerstrasse 26, 60594 Frankfurt am Main*

In Spain: Please write to *Penguin Books S. A., Bravo Murillo 19, 1° B, 28015 Madrid*

In Italy: Please write to *Penguin Italia s.r.l., Via Felice Casati 20, I–20124 Milano*

In France: Please write to *Penguin France S. A., 17 rue Lejeune, F–31000 Toulouse*

In Japan: Please write to *Penguin Books Japan, Ishikiribashi Building, 2–5–4, Suido, Bunkyo-ku, Tokyo 112*

In Greece: Please write to *Penguin Hellas Ltd, Dimocritou 3, GR–106 71 Athens*

In South Africa: Please write to *Longman Penguin Southern Africa (Pty) Ltd, Private Bag X08, Bertsham 2013*

BY THE SAME AUTHOR

Eva Fraser's Facial Workout

The remarkable facial exercise programme based on muscle physiology that reverses the signs of ageing – naturally

Many of our facial muscles are hardly used at all and as we grow older they slacken through underuse. Eva Fraser offers a unique step-by-step programme that allows you to improve the structure of your face dramatically and takes years off your appearance.

- Five workout programmes from basic to advanced – structured to build up facial muscles gradually and effectively
- Reduces wrinkles and improves facial contours
- Ten minutes a day will keep your face toned and fit
- Relieves stress and tension
- Massage routines to promote a healthy, vibrant skin
- Body workouts for general fitness

With special tips on hairstyling, make-up, vitamins and diet as well as basic exercises for health and beauty, *Eva Fraser's Facial Workout* is the key to recapturing your youthful looks.